# Waiting for Your Child

## To My Readers

I have for many years been privileged to help future mothers prepare for the great adventure of motherhood. This book contains a summary of my thinking along with answers to many of the questions expectant mothers have asked me. What can be more thrilling than to create a new life, experiencing week after week the subtle changes which take place while a child grows inside your body. This book, which is intended to prepare a couple for the birth of their child, is based on the medically-sound, practical prenatal courses so popular in Europe and the United States.

The main purpose of this book is to inform the future parents, especially the mother, of what can be expected during a pregnancy, thus eliminating any fear or uneasiness. It is also important for the future mother to learn to breathe properly. If she masters these two basic principles, every woman can deliver her child with a minimum of discomfort, either conscious or under anaesthetic. Having experimented with conscious deliveries on three occasions, I cannot forget the invaluable help of my husband during the time just before the baby was delivered. More and more, the future father has an important role to play at his wife's side — as much during the pregnancy as at the delivery.

I hope this book will add to your knowledge and make you excellent candidates for parenthood.

Y. P.-M.

Yvette Pratte Marchessault

# *Waiting for Your Child*

HABITEX BOOKS

- Cover design: JACQUES DESROSIERS
- Interior design: DONALD MORENCY
- Cover photo: RENÉ DELBUGUET
- Diagrams: Mme HÉLÈNE MAILLÉ-BLAIS
- Interior photos: M. AIMÉ DENIS
- In collaboration with: Dr. JEAN-LUC BEAULE (anaesthetist), Mme CHRISTIANE ST-PIERRE, Mme FRANÇOISE LALONDE, Mme LUCILLE DUSSAULT, Mme NICOLE BOURASSA, Mme FRANÇOISE D'ANJOU, Mme MONIQUE GAZAILLE and Mme LOUISE VÉZINA
- English language translation and production: AMPERSAND PUBLISHING SERVICES INC., Toronto

Habitex Books
955 Amherst Street
Montreal 132, P. Que.

Library of Congress Catalogue Card Number 73-85012

ISBN-0-88912-004-8

 2

*Bibliothèque nationale du Québec*
*Dépôt légal — 3e trimestre 1973*

# Table of Contents

# Glossary of Terms

**Abdominal girdle:** a belt of elastic tissue which supports the abdominal muscles.

**Albuminuria:** the presence of albumen in the urine.

**Amniotic fluid:** the fluid which completely surrounds the fetus in the uterus.

**Anorexia:** lack of appetite or inability to eat.

**Areolae:** the brownish rings of skin of the breast surrounding the nipple.

**Bulimia:** feeling of excessive hunger, particularly for specific foods; a strong craving for food.

**Colostrum:** the fluid secreted by the breasts before childbirth and a few days before milk appears.

**Contraction:** a spontaneous tightening of the muscles of the uterus which occurs during the last months of pregnancy and just prior to delivery.

**Dilation:** a widening of the cervix as a result of uterine contractions. It is measured in centimeters.

**Diuresis:** increased discharge of urine.

**Diuretic:** a drug which causes increased urination.

**Dystocia:** a difficult labor.

**Eclampsia:** the most severe stage of an acute toximia of pregnancy. It is one of the gravest complications that can arise in pregnancy.

**Edema:** a swelling of the extremities, particularly of the feet and hands due to the storage of large quantities of water by the tissues.

**Embryo:** the term applied to an organism during the first two to three months of its intra-uterine development.

**Episiotomy:** a surgical operation involving an incision of the perineum muscle (vulva) to facilitate delivery of the fetus.

**Eructation:** belching; stomach gas.

**Foetoscope:** an instrument similar to a stethoscope but designed specifically to enable one to hear a fetus' heartbeat through the mother's abdominal wall.

**Fetus:** the term applied to a developing organism during its intra-uterine existence after approximately its second to third month of life.

**Hydramnios:** the presence of an excessive amount of amniotic fluid.

**Hypertension:** high blood pressure.

**Hyperthyroid:** an over-active functioning of the thyroid gland.

**Inappetence:** lack of appetite.

**Lanugo:** a downy hair which covers the entire body of the fetus during much of its intra-uterine life.

**Ligaments:** white fibrous bands of tissue usually serving to connect bones, hold vital organs in place, etc.

**Meconium:** a tarry fecal material in the intestines of the fetus during its intra-uterine development.

**Menopause:** the period of permanent cessation of menstruation usually occurring between the ages of 45 and 50.

**Membranes:** the double sac of tissue surrounding the fetus, containing the amniotic fluid and serving to protect the organism from infection.

**Micturition:** urination.

**Montgomery's**
**Tubercules:** small protuberances located in the areolae around the nipples.

**Multigravida:** a woman who is in her second or any subsequent pregnancy.

**Parturient:** a woman in labor.

**Parturition:** the act of bringing forth young; childbirth.

**Placenta:** the spongy mass adhering to the wall of the uterus by one surface, known as the maternal surface, and from which the umbilical cord emerges. The placenta serves as an intermediate connection along with the umbilical cord between the mother and child.

**Placenta previa:** a poor positioning of the placenta with the result that the placenta either partially or completely covers the opening from the uterus. This condition usually requires a Caesarian.

**Polyuria:** the passing of an excessive amount of urine.

**Post-partum:** the period following childbirth.

**Post-partum
bleeding:** a loss of blood from the birth canal following delivery of a baby and discharge of its placenta. It may be a heavy flow for the first two days following birth but reduces steadily during the following two to four weeks.

**Post-partum
contractions:** uterine contractions which may take place after delivery and which are related to expulsion of the placenta.

**Primigravida:** a woman who is pregnant for the first time.

**Prolapse:** the fall of an organ (such as the uterus or the bladder).

**Pruritus:** itching; tingling.

**Sebum:** see vernix caseosa.

**Stretch-marks:** lines appearing on the abdomen and breasts during and after pregnancy because of stretching of the elastic tissues in the skin.

**Stethoscope:** an instrument used by a physician which enables him to listen to a patient's heartbeat.

**Toxemia of Pregnancy:** poisoning of the organism by self-produced toxins (poisons) leading to convulsions.

**Umbilical cord:** a twisted cord made up of three blood vessels (one vein and two arteries) extending from the placenta to the abdomen of the fetus. Its purpose is to carry oxygen and nourishment to the fetus which is required for its development.

**Uterus:** also known as the womb, this is the organ in which the fetus develops and from which menstruation occurs. It is a muscular structure situated in the pelvic cavity and during pregnancy contains the fetus, placenta, umbilical cord and the amniotic fluid.

**Vernix Caseosa:** a greasy white substance which covers the body of the baby at birth. Also referred to as sebum.

I dedicate this book to my three daughters, Marie-France, Marie-Claude and Lyne, who, I hope, will one day know the great joy of giving birth to a child. I cannot overlook the help and encouragement of my husband who took such good care of me through each of the three pregnancies. I especially appreciate the comfort which his presence at my side through the deliveries gave me, and his lavish encouragement which never ceased throughout those unforgettable hours.

**Y. P.-M.**

# Chapter I

## Discovering You're Pregnant

The discovery that you are pregnant is one of the most important moments in a woman's life. This book is intended to acquaint you with the dramatic changes which take place in a woman's body when she is pregnant. If you are expecting your first child, what follows here should help you to anticipate with joy an experience that, although timeless, is always unique. If you have other children, perhaps this book will add to your knowledge and increase your enjoyment of that time of waiting. Discuss the material with your husband, particularly the references addressed to him.

## Some of the Signs of Pregnancy

**Changes in the menstrual cycle** — normally, this means missing a period or the absence of menstruation altogether. (Amenorrhea is the medical term for this.) In some cases, you may be pregnant and still have a period. It is usually different, however, in that it is of longer duration, the flow may be heavier and its appearance unlike the usual.

**Drowziness** — especially after meals. Tiredness and mild fatigue are also frequent symptoms.

**Morning sickness** — a feeling of nausea upon waking which may be followed by vomiting. Occasionally, nausea during the day (including vomiting) may also occur.

**Changes in appetite** — these may include a loss of appetite, a distaste for certain foods, excessive hunger or a pronounced craving for certain foods.

**Increased sensitivity to odors** — certain odors may become unbearable.

**Increased salivation** — a marked increase in the secretion of saliva.

**Stomach pains** — gas, swelling and discomfort.

**Positive lab test** — 12 days or more after a missed period. There are at least two new tests now on the market which you can administer yourself at home. These may indicate the beginning of a pregnancy as early as four days after your period should normally have begun.

**Changes in disposition** — occasional irritability and other changes in your usual behaviour patterns.

**Frequent urination** — usually occurs for a few weeks at the beginning of pregnancy and again during the ninth month. This happens as a result of the increased flow of blood in the abdomen and pelvic region and the enlargement of the uterus which exerts pressure on the bladder.

**Changes in the breasts** — toward the end of the first month, some tingling and a certain heaviness may be felt in the breasts as they become more sensitive. This is a sign that they are being prepared for nursing. The areola, the brown part surrounding the nipple, takes on a darker colour and increases in size while the Montgomery tubercules ( small protuberences around the nipple) become more prominent. (See Diagram 1)

**Constipation** — or sometimes diarrhoea.

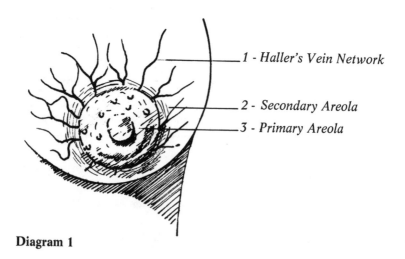

1 - *Haller's Vein Network*

2 - *Secondary Areola*

3 - *Primary Areola*

**Diagram 1**

# Choosing Your Doctor

## Family Doctor or Specialist?

**The family doctor** or general practitioner is one who has had at least five years of university training followed by an internship in a hospital. As a family doctor, he is generally well-acquainted with his patients since he may be consulted frequently by an entire family.

**The obstetrician** is a doctor who specializes in the branch of medicine called obstetrics. He is particularly concerned with childbirth and caring for and treating women in or in connection with childbirth. As a specialist, he is experienced and has been specifically trained to deal with any possible complication related to childbirth.

**The obstetrician-gynecologist** is a doctor who specializes in two areas — obstetrics and gynecology. (The latter is the branch of medicine which deals with the functions and diseases peculiar to women — particularly of the reproductive system.) A Caesarian delivery is necessarily performed by an obstetrician-gynecologist.

**Clinics** are usually formed by several doctors who combine their talents and work together in a group practice. If you attend a clinic regularly, you will no doubt see more than one doctor during the course of your pregnancy. Having more than one doctor offers an advantage, particularly if there are complications, because each of them is familiar with your case and they can consult on it. You can also be sure that one of them will be in attendance when your baby is delivered. A disadvantage of the clinic arrangement is that you cannot be certain of seeing the same doctor on every visit.

If you wish to have natural childbirth, you should discuss your intention with your doctor on your first visit. He will be able to advise you accordingly. You should know in advance, however, that many physicians do not favour this method of delivery.

You will also want to learn the name of the hospital the

13

doctor is associated with and where you can expect to have your child delivered. Having this information will help you to make your choice of a physician.

## Your First Visit to the Doctor

Although you may have some of the symptoms described earlier, your first visit to the doctor is important because he will confirm whether or not you are pregnant. Having determined that you are, you can ask him questions and discuss openly with him any concerns you may have. Certain knowledge and correct information should then permit you to begin your pregnancy calmly and serenely.

It is not unusual to feel a little tense during your first visit, but try to relax and do your best to answer the doctor's questions fully. You should also remember that the doctor has attended many women in the same circumstances and therefore you should not feel uneasy about the examination.

It is a good idea to have your husband accompany you on your first visit. It is a convenient time for him to meet your doctor; the doctor, in turn, can use the opportunity to explain to you both the nature of pregnancy and the physical changes which will take place in your body over the next several months. (Illust. 1)

Your doctor will tell you that pregnancy is a normal condition — it is not an illness — and that many women feel happiest and best when they are pregnant.

## When Will Your Baby be Born?

A normal pregnancy usually lasts 38 weeks. However, it can vary from one pregnancy to another as much as 15 days more or less. To calculate the approximate birth date of your child, add 9 months and 7 days to the starting date of your last period or, alternatively, take the starting date of your last period, add 7 days then subtract 3 months. For example, if your last period began on June 20th, your baby should be born about March 27th. (June 20th + 7 days = June 27 − 3 months = March 27th.)

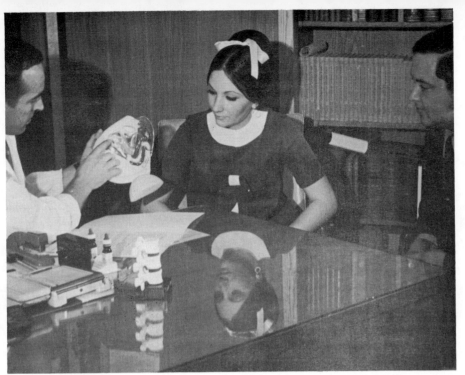

**Illust. 1**

You can calculate the date of your probable delivery more precisely by referring to the table on page 28.

Your doctor or his nurse will take your blood pressure on each of your regular visits to his office. (Illust. 2) This is a convenient time to tell him about your problems, worries or other concerns. To save time, it is a good idea to make a list of your questions between visits so that you can discuss them with your doctor when you see him.

At the beginning of your pregnancy, one visit each month is usually sufficient. Toward the end, your doctor will want to see you more frequently — probably once every two weeks.

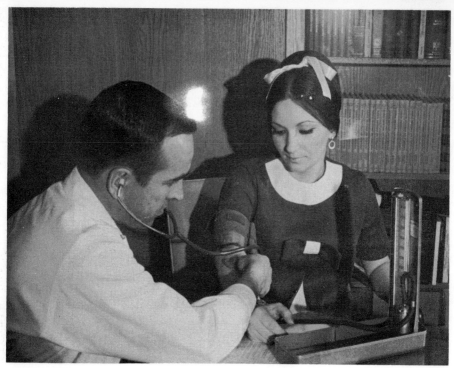

**Illust. 2**

Your weight during pregnancy is very important and your doctor will watch it carefully. (Illust. 3) Over the nine-month period, you may add from 18 to 24 pounds to your normal weight.

The weight increase breaks down as follows:

| | |
|---|---|
| Weight of average baby | 7 pounds |
| Placenta | 1 to 1½ pounds |
| Amniotic fluid or the waters | 2 pounds |
| Enlargement of the uterus | 2 pounds |
| Enlargement of the breasts | 2 to 3 pounds |
| Water retention | 4 pounds |
| Increased volume of blood | 2 pounds |
| Total | 20 to 22 pounds |

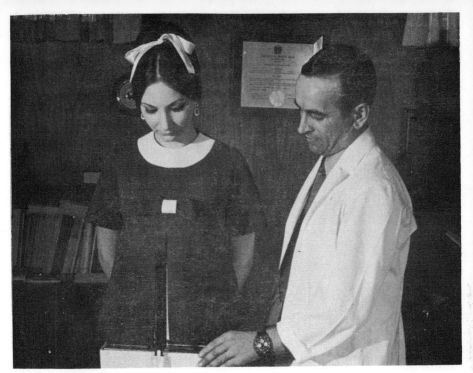

**Illust. 3**

It should be noted that the figures provided here are average estimates only. A woman carrying twins — each weighing 5 to 6 pounds — can expect to gain more than 20 pounds. A slight woman may also gain substantially — up to 30 pounds — during her pregnancy, hoping to retain some of the weight afterwards. A woman who is already over her normal weight should follow a sensible diet and exercise regularly in order to avoid further unnecessary weight gain. She will be happy with her svelte figure after the child is born!

During the first 3 months, there is usually little weight gain, indeed, some women even lose weight. Thereafter, the weight gain is usually between one-half to three-quarters of a pound each week, or between 2 and 3 pounds a month. A few days before delivery you may lose 2 to 3 pounds. This loss of weight is caused by the elimination of fluids.

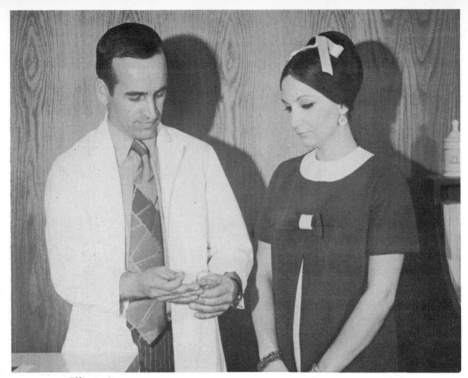

**Illust. 4**

Immediately after delivery you will lose 11 to 12 pounds. The excess will disappear during the following few weeks so that by the time you make your first postnatal visit to the doctor (after your period returns to normal, usually from 40 to 70 days after delivery) you should have returned to your normal weight.

On your regular monthly prenatal visits to the doctor, you will be asked to bring a morning urine sample which will be tested for sugar or albumin. (Illust. 4) This test, taken regularly, will avoid serious complications like toxemia. Fortunately, this condition occurs very rarely today because it can be diagnosed quickly and appropriate measures taken to prevent it.

Swollen ankles are another sign of possible trouble. (Illust. 5) This condition (edema) is usually caused by excessive water retention, and is related to your diet. Some doctors

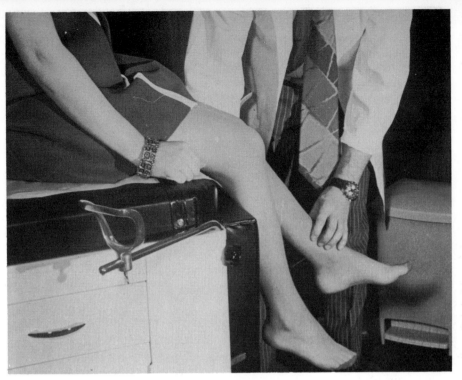

**Illust. 5**

prescribe a salt-free diet beginning in the fourth month as a matter of course in order to avoid this problem. If the edema persists, your doctor may prescribe a diuretic (a drug which causes increased urination). This will reduce swelling of the feet and ankles by reducing the water being held in the tissues. Diuretics should be taken **only** under medical supervision.

Your doctor must know the state of your general health in order to detect any problem which might influence the successful progress of your pregnancy. He will pay particular attention to your heart and lungs, and will listen carefully to your heartbeat and breathing through his stethescope. (Iillust. 6)

Your doctor will measure the height of your uterus in order to calculate the approximate stage of your pregnancy. (Illust. 7) He will also measure your pelvis to ensure that there are

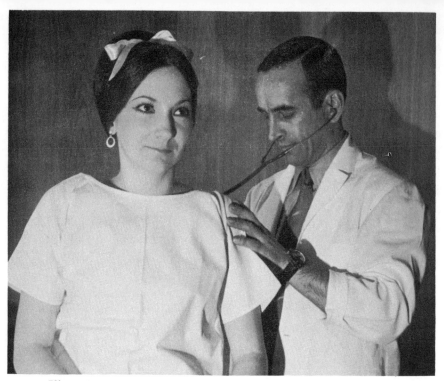

Illust. 6

Illust. 7

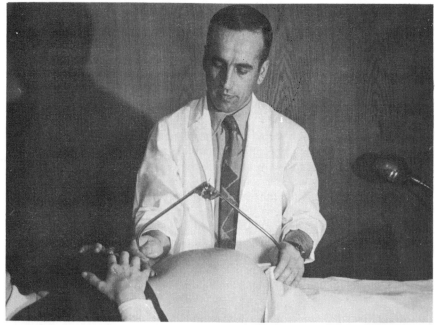

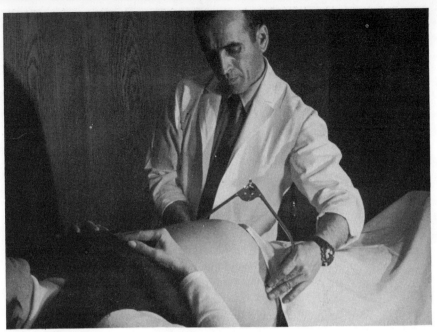

**Illust. 8**

no problems which might preclude a normal delivery. (Illust. 8)

Listening to the heartbeat of the fetus for the first time is a memorable experience. The doctor can hear it through his foetoscope (Illust. 9) about the fifth or sixth month. The rate is quick — from 140 to 160 beats per minute. If there are twins, two heartbeats may be heard. There is an old wives' tale that says if the baby's heatbeat is 140 it will be a boy, but if it is 160 it will be a girl. There is a 50% chance of error in this theory, however!

The first movements of the fetus are felt around the four-month point on the average — usually 3½ months for a woman who has been pregnant before and 4½ months for a first pregnancy. It is also normal for some new mothers-to-be to feel no movement at all until the fifth month.

When it happens for the first time, the sensation is rather like having butterflies in your stomach.

21

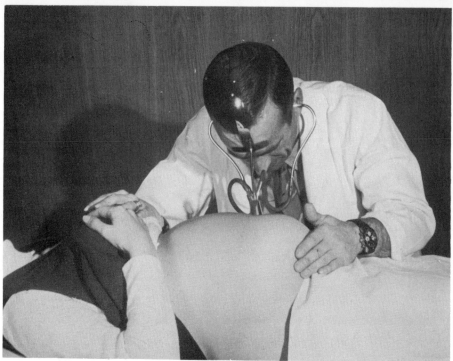

**Illust. 9**

When you get used to these movements, you will feel very distinct little kicks. By standing in front of a mirror you can occasionally see them. The fetus makes approximately 200 movements in a day. Although you will not feel all of them, they may be particularly noticeable when you are relaxed — sitting or lying down. Your baby will take the opportunity to adjust his position when you are relaxed because it is then easier for him to move.

It is notable that after practicing the deep breathing exercises recommended in most prenatal classes, many expectant mothers say their babies move much more frequently. This is undoubtedly due to the increased amount of oxygen which the babies are receiving.

Occasionally, an expectant mother will worry if she does not experience "signs of life" every day. Such concern is usually unnecessary, although if, after the sixth month, no movement

22

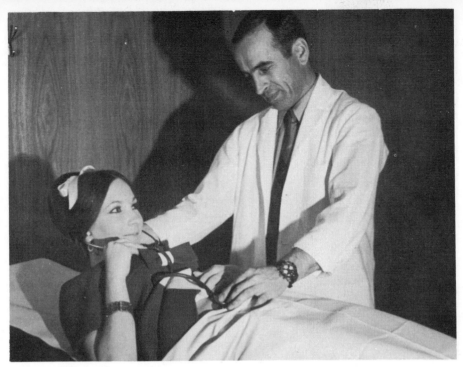

**Illust. 10**

is felt for more than three days, you should get in touch with your doctor.

Your doctor will let you listen to your baby's heart with his stethescope. (Illust. 10) At first, the sound may be vague, but by being attentive and blocking out any surrounding noise, you should be able to hear a distinct "thump-thump". This is an experience no mother will ever forget.

In some cases, the doctor cannot hear the baby's heartbeat because of the position of the placenta which muffles the sound. In such cases the doctor will listen for placental breathing.

Your husband will also have an opportunity to hear the heartbeat of the child developing within you through the doctor's foetoscope. (Illust. 11) He can hear it without this instrument, however, by placing his ear on your abdomen a few inches to the left of your navel. If no sound is heard,

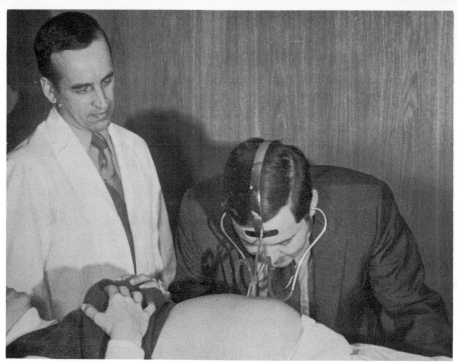

**Illust. 11**

have him move his head around until a heartbeat can be heard.

About six weeks after conception, a gynaecological examination is very important in diagnosing a pregnancy. Although many women are inclined to feel uneasy about it, there is really nothing to worry about. The examination is simple and every precaution will be taken to preserve your modesty. You should try to relax; go completely limp if possible. If you take a deep breath when the doctor inserts his fingers into the vagina, you will feel absolutely nothing.

During your pregnancy, the uterus will undergo dramatic change. It will change its triangular shape and become round; it will toughen and its consistency will change; it will change its position and grow larger. At conception, the uterus is approximately the size and shape of a pear; after six weeks it enlarges to the size of a tangerine; by the eighth

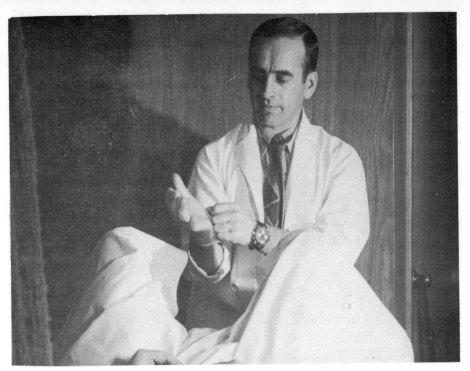

**Illust. 12**

week it is approximately the size of a large orange. The doctor will determine the position of the uterus by feeling the abdomen. (Illust. 13)

Early in your pregnancy, you will probably have a blood test in order to determine your blood type and to evaluate the quality of your hemoglobin. This blood test will also indicate if you have any infection or other blood abnormalities.

Your doctor may give you a prescription for some medication which you will have filled by a pharmacist. (Illust. 14) This might include calcium and vitamins which are especially important for you to take at this time. **Do not take any other medicines without the permission of your doctor.**

You should pay particular attention to your teeth while you are pregnant. If you have any cavities, you should have them filled. In any case, you should make a point of visiting your

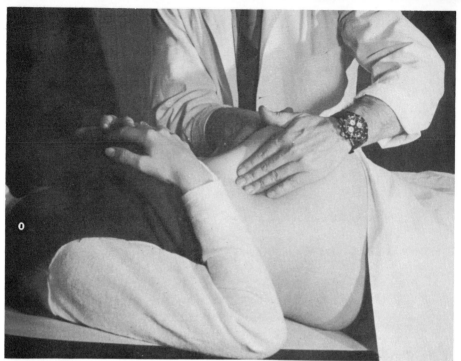

Illust. 13

Illust. 14

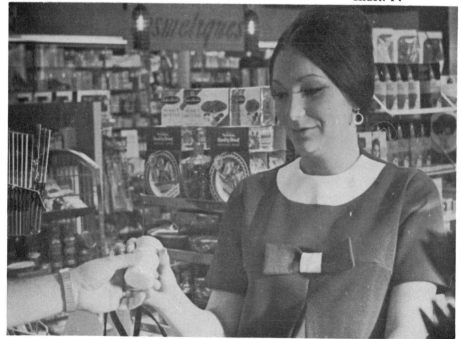

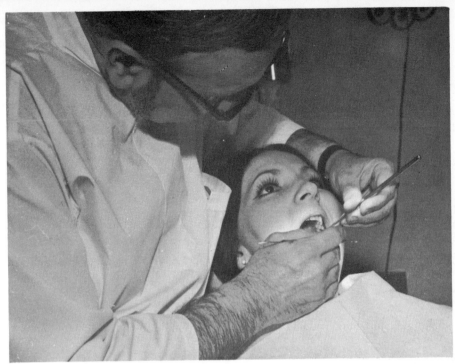

**Illust. 15**

dentist for a check-up. Dental hygiene is also very important and you should brush your teeth after every meal — preferably within 20 minutes because it is during this period immediately after eating that acid levels in the mouth are highest and cavities are most likely to begin.

Your doctor will prescribe a surplus of calcium for you during the first months of your pregnancy in order to ensure that your developing fetus has sufficient quantities available for building strong bones and teeth. This is very important because it is during the first months of intre-uterine life that your baby develops the basis for sound bones and teeth which will be with him for the rest of his life. You should, therefore, be especially careful to avoid a calcium deficiency.

# GESTATION CALENDAR

| Start | 1 | 2 | 3 | 4 | 5 | 6 | 7 | 8 | 9 | 10 | 11 | 12 | 13 | 14 | 15 | 16 | 17 | 18 | 19 | 20 | 21 | 22 | 23 | 24 | 25 | 26 | 27 | 28 | 29 | 30 | 31 | End |
|---|---|---|---|---|---|---|---|---|---|---|---|---|---|---|---|---|---|---|---|---|---|---|---|---|---|---|---|---|---|---|---|---|
| **JANUARY** | 1 | 2 | 3 | 4 | 5 | 6 | 7 | 8 | 9 | 10 | 11 | 12 | 13 | 14 | 15 | 16 | 17 | 18 | 19 | 20 | 21 | 22 | 23 | 24 | 25 | 26 | 27 | 28 | 29 | 30 | 31 | **JANUARY** |
| **MAY** | 21 | 22 | 23 | 24 | 25 | 26 | 27 | 28 | 29 | 30 | 31 | 1 | 2 | 3 | 4 | 5 | 6 | 7 | 8 | 9 | 10 | 11 | 12 | 13 | 14 | 15 | 16 | 17 | 18 | 19 | 20 | **JUNE** |
| **OCTOBER** | 8 | 9 | 10 | 11 | 12 | 13 | 14 | 15 | 16 | 17 | 18 | 19 | 20 | 21 | 22 | 23 | 24 | 25 | 26 | 27 | 28 | 29 | 30 | 31 | 1 | 2 | 3 | 4 | 5 | 6 | 7 | **NOVEMBER** |
| **FEBRUARY** | 1 | 2 | 3 | 4 | 5 | 6 | 7 | 8 | 9 | 10 | 11 | 12 | 13 | 14 | 15 | 16 | 17 | 18 | 19 | 20 | 21 | 22 | 23 | 24 | 25 | 26 | 27 | 28 | — | — | — | **FEBRUARY** |
| **JUNE** | 21 | 22 | 23 | 24 | 25 | 26 | 27 | 28 | 29 | 30 | 1 | 2 | 3 | 4 | 5 | 6 | 7 | 8 | 9 | 10 | 11 | 12 | 13 | 14 | 15 | 16 | 17 | 18 | — | — | — | **JULY** |
| **NOVEMBER** | 8 | 9 | 10 | 11 | 12 | 13 | 14 | 15 | 16 | 17 | 18 | 19 | 20 | 21 | 22 | 23 | 24 | 25 | 26 | 27 | 28 | 29 | 30 | 1 | 2 | 3 | 4 | 5 | — | — | — | **DECEMBER** |
| **MARCH** | 1 | 2 | 3 | 4 | 5 | 6 | 7 | 8 | 9 | 10 | 11 | 12 | 13 | 14 | 15 | 16 | 17 | 18 | 19 | 20 | 21 | 22 | 23 | 24 | 25 | 26 | 27 | 28 | 29 | 30 | 31 | **MARCH** |
| **JULY** | 19 | 20 | 21 | 22 | 23 | 24 | 25 | 26 | 27 | 28 | 29 | 30 | 31 | 1 | 2 | 3 | 4 | 5 | 6 | 7 | 8 | 9 | 10 | 11 | 12 | 13 | 14 | 15 | 16 | 17 | 18 | **AUGUST** |
| **DECEMBER** | 6 | 7 | 8 | 9 | 10 | 11 | 12 | 13 | 14 | 15 | 16 | 17 | 18 | 19 | 20 | 21 | 22 | 23 | 24 | 25 | 26 | 27 | 28 | 29 | 30 | 31 | 1 | 2 | 3 | 4 | 5 | **JANUARY** |
| **APRIL** | 1 | 2 | 3 | 4 | 5 | 6 | 7 | 8 | 9 | 10 | 11 | 12 | 13 | 14 | 15 | 16 | 17 | 18 | 19 | 20 | 21 | 22 | 23 | 24 | 25 | 26 | 27 | 28 | 29 | 30 | — | **APRIL** |
| **AUGUST** | 19 | 20 | 21 | 22 | 23 | 24 | 25 | 26 | 27 | 28 | 29 | 30 | 31 | 1 | 2 | 3 | 4 | 5 | 6 | 7 | 8 | 9 | 10 | 11 | 12 | 13 | 14 | 15 | 16 | 17 | — | **SEPTEMBER** |
| **JANUARY** | 6 | 7 | 8 | 9 | 10 | 11 | 12 | 13 | 14 | 15 | 16 | 17 | 18 | 19 | 20 | 21 | 22 | 23 | 24 | 25 | 26 | 27 | 28 | 29 | 30 | 31 | 1 | 2 | 3 | 4 | — | **FEBRUARY** |
| **MAY** | 1 | 2 | 3 | 4 | 5 | 6 | 7 | 8 | 9 | 10 | 11 | 12 | 13 | 14 | 15 | 16 | 17 | 18 | 19 | 20 | 21 | 22 | 23 | 24 | 25 | 26 | 27 | 28 | 29 | 30 | 31 | **MAY** |
| **SEPTEMBER** | 18 | 19 | 20 | 21 | 22 | 23 | 24 | 25 | 26 | 27 | 28 | 29 | 30 | 1 | 2 | 3 | 4 | 5 | 6 | 7 | 8 | 9 | 10 | 11 | 12 | 13 | 14 | 15 | 16 | 17 | 18 | **OCTOBER** |
| **FEBRUARY** | 5 | 6 | 7 | 8 | 9 | 10 | 11 | 12 | 13 | 14 | 15 | 16 | 17 | 18 | 19 | 20 | 21 | 22 | 23 | 24 | 25 | 26 | 27 | 28 | 1 | 2 | 3 | 4 | 5 | 6 | 7 | **MARCH** |
| **JUNE** | 1 | 2 | 3 | 4 | 5 | 6 | 7 | 8 | 9 | 10 | 11 | 12 | 13 | 14 | 15 | 16 | 17 | 18 | 19 | 20 | 21 | 22 | 23 | 24 | 25 | 26 | 27 | 28 | 29 | 30 | — | **JUNE** |
| **OCTOBER** | 19 | 20 | 21 | 22 | 23 | 24 | 25 | 26 | 27 | 28 | 29 | 30 | 31 | 1 | 2 | 3 | 4 | 5 | 6 | 7 | 8 | 9 | 10 | 11 | 12 | 13 | 14 | 15 | 16 | 17 | — | **NOVEMBER** |
| **MARCH** | 8 | 9 | 10 | 11 | 12 | 13 | 14 | 15 | 16 | 17 | 18 | 19 | 20 | 21 | 22 | 23 | 24 | 25 | 26 | 27 | 28 | 29 | 30 | 31 | 1 | 2 | 3 | 4 | 5 | 6 | — | **APRIL** |
| **JULY** | 1 | 2 | 3 | 4 | 5 | 6 | 7 | 8 | 9 | 10 | 11 | 12 | 13 | 14 | 15 | 16 | 17 | 18 | 19 | 20 | 21 | 22 | 23 | 24 | 25 | 26 | 27 | 28 | 29 | 30 | 31 | **JULY** |
| **NOVEMBER** | 18 | 19 | 20 | 21 | 22 | 23 | 24 | 25 | 26 | 27 | 28 | 29 | 30 | 1 | 2 | 3 | 4 | 5 | 6 | 7 | 8 | 9 | 10 | 11 | 12 | 13 | 14 | 15 | 16 | 17 | 18 | **DECEMBER** |
| **APRIL** | 7 | 8 | 9 | 10 | 11 | 12 | 13 | 14 | 15 | 16 | 17 | 18 | 19 | 20 | 21 | 22 | 23 | 24 | 25 | 26 | 27 | 28 | 29 | 30 | 1 | 2 | 3 | 4 | 5 | 6 | 7 | **MAY** |
| **AUGUST** | 1 | 2 | 3 | 4 | 5 | 6 | 7 | 8 | 9 | 10 | 11 | 12 | 13 | 14 | 15 | 16 | 17 | 18 | 19 | 20 | 21 | 22 | 23 | 24 | 25 | 26 | 27 | 28 | 29 | 30 | 31 | **AUGUST** |
| **DECEMBER** | 19 | 20 | 21 | 22 | 23 | 24 | 25 | 26 | 27 | 28 | 29 | 30 | 31 | 1 | 2 | 3 | 4 | 5 | 6 | 7 | 8 | 9 | 10 | 11 | 12 | 13 | 14 | 15 | 16 | 17 | 18 | **JANUARY** |
| **MAY** | 8 | 9 | 10 | 11 | 12 | 13 | 14 | 15 | 16 | 17 | 18 | 19 | 20 | 21 | 22 | 23 | 24 | 25 | 26 | 27 | 28 | 29 | 30 | 31 | 1 | 2 | 3 | 4 | 5 | 6 | 7 | **JUNE** |
| **SEPTEMBER** | 1 | 2 | 3 | 4 | 5 | 6 | 7 | 8 | 9 | 10 | 11 | 12 | 13 | 14 | 15 | 16 | 17 | 18 | 19 | 20 | 21 | 22 | 23 | 24 | 25 | 26 | 27 | 28 | 29 | 30 | — | **SEPTEMBER** |
| **JANUARY** | 19 | 20 | 21 | 22 | 23 | 24 | 25 | 26 | 27 | 28 | 29 | 30 | 31 | 1 | 2 | 3 | 4 | 5 | 6 | 7 | 8 | 9 | 10 | 11 | 12 | 13 | 14 | 15 | 16 | 17 | — | **FEBRUARY** |
| **JUNE** | 8 | 9 | 10 | 11 | 12 | 13 | 14 | 15 | 16 | 17 | 18 | 19 | 20 | 21 | 22 | 23 | 24 | 25 | 26 | 27 | 28 | 29 | 30 | 1 | 2 | 3 | 4 | 5 | 6 | 7 | — | **JULY** |
| **OCTOBER** | 1 | 2 | 3 | 4 | 5 | 6 | 7 | 8 | 9 | 10 | 11 | 12 | 13 | 14 | 15 | 16 | 17 | 18 | 19 | 20 | 21 | 22 | 23 | 24 | 25 | 26 | 27 | 28 | 29 | 30 | 31 | **OCTOBER** |
| **FEBRUARY** | 18 | 19 | 20 | 21 | 22 | 23 | 24 | 25 | 26 | 27 | 28 | 1 | 2 | 3 | 4 | 5 | 6 | 7 | 8 | 9 | 10 | 11 | 12 | 13 | 14 | 15 | 16 | 17 | 18 | 19 | 20 | **MARCH** |
| **JULY** | 8 | 9 | 10 | 11 | 12 | 13 | 14 | 15 | 16 | 17 | 18 | 19 | 20 | 21 | 22 | 23 | 24 | 25 | 26 | 27 | 28 | 29 | 30 | 31 | 1 | 2 | 3 | 4 | 5 | 6 | 7 | **AUGUST** |
| **NOVEMBER** | 1 | 2 | 3 | 4 | 5 | 6 | 7 | 8 | 9 | 10 | 11 | 12 | 13 | 14 | 15 | 16 | 17 | 18 | 19 | 20 | 21 | 22 | 23 | 24 | 25 | 26 | 27 | 28 | 29 | 30 | — | **NOVEMBER** |
| **MARCH** | 21 | 22 | 23 | 24 | 25 | 26 | 27 | 28 | 29 | 30 | 31 | 1 | 2 | 3 | 4 | 5 | 6 | 7 | 8 | 9 | 10 | 11 | 12 | 13 | 14 | 15 | 16 | 17 | 18 | 19 | — | **APRIL** |
| **AUGUST** | 8 | 9 | 10 | 11 | 12 | 13 | 14 | 15 | 16 | 17 | 18 | 19 | 20 | 21 | 22 | 23 | 24 | 25 | 26 | 27 | 28 | 29 | 30 | 31 | 1 | 2 | 3 | 4 | 5 | 6 | — | **SEPTEMBER** |
| **DECEMBER** | 1 | 2 | 3 | 4 | 5 | 6 | 7 | 8 | 9 | 10 | 11 | 12 | 13 | 14 | 15 | 16 | 17 | 18 | 19 | 20 | 21 | 22 | 23 | 24 | 25 | 26 | 27 | 28 | 29 | 30 | 31 | **DECEMBER** |
| **APRIL** | 20 | 21 | 22 | 23 | 24 | 25 | 26 | 27 | 28 | 29 | 30 | 1 | 2 | 3 | 4 | 5 | 6 | 7 | 8 | 9 | 10 | 11 | 12 | 13 | 14 | 15 | 16 | 17 | 18 | 19 | 20 | **MAY** |
| **SEPTEMBER** | 7 | 8 | 9 | 10 | 11 | 12 | 13 | 14 | 15 | 16 | 17 | 18 | 19 | 20 | 21 | 22 | 23 | 24 | 25 | 26 | 27 | 28 | 29 | 30 | 1 | 2 | 3 | 4 | 5 | 6 | 7 | **OCTOBER** |

On the top line of each section, find the date of the first day of your last period. The date immediately below is the approximate date when the first movement of the fetus may be felt. The date on the third line of the section is the approximate date of delivery.

# Chapter II

## Adapting to the Changes in your Body

It is especially important for the mother-to-be to adopt a positive attitude toward this exciting adventure. Waiting for a child to be born is a creative, super-natural experience even though much of what happens to you is on a natural plane. For example, the thrill of feeling the baby's first movements will sometimes be off-set by day-to-day physical problems.

Pregnancy can be roughly divided into three periods:

**First Trimester**   Period of Adaptation — 1st, 2nd and 3rd months. This is the period when risk of miscarriage is most probable.

**Second Trimester**   Period of Equilibrium — 4th, 5th and 6th months. This is the period when the body of the future mother seems perfectly adapted to accommodating the fetus. The uterus is not yet large enough to be troublesome and the risk of miscarriage is reduced. This is probably the easiest time of the pregnancy.

**Third Trimester**   Period of rest — 7th, 8th and 9th months. This is the period during which the uterus increases in size and applies pressure on the other vital organs. This is the time when problems may occur.

## Some Common Problems of Pregnancy

**Nausea**   Approximately 50% of pregnant women experience some symptoms of nausea.

Nausea in the morning, or "morning sickness" is caused by the movement of the empty stomach as you get up and begin moving around. A feeling of nausea may be followed by vomiting of mucus or bile.

An effective way to prevent morning sickness is to place some unsalted soda crackers and a glass of tomato juice or milk beside your bed before retiring. Eat these when you wake up and stay quiet for another 15 minutes, then get up slowly and wait a further half-hour before breakfast.

In case of nausea or vomiting between meals, try having smaller, more frequent meals, instead of three larger ones and lie down with your legs raised for ten minutes after eating.

**Heartburn**  A burning sensation in the stomach, usually caused by overeating.

This can be dealt with by eliminating fats and rich foods from your diet as far as possible. It is not a good idea to take bicarbonate of soda or commercial preparations without your doctor's permission. If you are especially bothered by heartburn, avoid foods such as cabbage, beans, onions and turnips, and if it persists, your doctor will prescribe a medication.

**Constipation**  This is caused by the enlargement of the uterus which applies pressure on the intestinal tract and prevents it from functioning normally.

Eat plenty of green vegetables and fruits, especially prunes and figs. Substitute whole wheat bread for white and unrefined brown sugar for white. Drink plenty of fresh fruit juices and, if you have a blender, puré vegetables and drink the juice. Pure honey and brewer's yeast will also help prevent constipation. Be sure to do your prenatal exercises every day and walking in the fresh air is especially good. Never use an enema or take a laxative without consulting your doctor.

**Diarrhea**  Again, do not take any medication. If it persists, call your doctor. It could be an intestinal infection.

**Urinary Discomfort**  This is also caused by the enlarged uterus exerting pressure on the bladder. It is usually most noticeable during the first and last months of pregnancy.

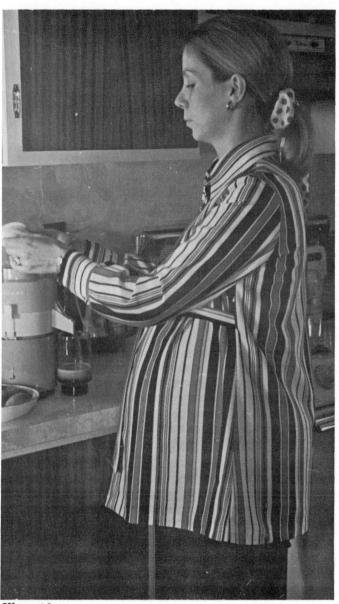

Illust. 16

Limit your fluid intake especially during the evening, so that you will not have to get up during the night. It is not unusual to lose control of the bladder while sneezing, coughing or performing some physical task.

**Faintness and/or Dizziness**  Lie down for a few minutes with your feet elevated so the blood runs to your head. Be sure to tell your doctor about any dizzy or fainting spells, it could be a sign of anemia.

**Shortness of Breath**  As the uterus grows, it pushes the abdomen against the thorax, thus reducing the volume of air you can hold in your chest. Avoid climbing stairs too quickly and breathe more rapidly while doing so. Take two or three deep breaths on reaching the top.

**Headaches**  Many pregnant women suffer from headaches. If they persist, consult your doctor.

**Leg and Foot Cramps**  These occur frequently. They could be caused by a calcium deficiency or a lack of vitamin B.

Be sure that you are taking the proper amount of calcium and vitamins prescribed by your doctor. Most leg and foot cramps occur at night. The best way to cure them is to get out of bed and walk around until they disappear. Avoid stretching when you first wake up in the morning.

**Lumbago**  Pain in the lumbar (lower or "small" of the back) region. This may occur around the fifth month of pregnancy and is due to the fact that the ligaments which attach the bones of the pelvis are gradually slackening. Another very frequent cause of lumbago is that the future mother has too great a tendency to hollow the lumbar region to counterbalance the weight of the uterus which pulls her forward. The enlarged uterus is not sufficiently supported my strong muscles and moves too far forward, which increases the forward curvature of the spine and therefore provokes the lumbar pain. See Chapter III for exercises which will strengthen the muscles of the lower back

**Insomnia** This is a common problem during the last few months of pregnancy. The movements of the fetus are stronger and more frequent and you may be troubled with back pain.

Here are some suggestions which may help you to sleep:

• Make your evening meal a light one so that you can have a snack before retiring.

• Take a short walk before going to bed.

• If you do your prenatal and breathing exercises just before bedtime, they will help you to relax.

• Take a warm bath before going to bed.

• Avoid stimulants such as coffee and tea, especially in the evening.

• When you get into bed, try to relax all your muscles, close your eyes, let your head fall back and yawn, opening your mouth as wide as possible.

• Try munching an apple.

If these methods do not work, as your doctor for a light sedative, but **never** take barbiturates without his authorization.

**White Discharge** This is frequent in pregnant women, and more abundant in the ninth month. It is due to the congestion of the genital organs. If it is accompanied by itching and burning, tell your doctor and he will prescribe medication.

**Varicose Veins** The enlarged uterus puts pressure on the veins through which the blood from the legs returns to the heart. The constriction of these veins hampers the circulation and the veins become larger, often causing varicose veins and/or hemorrhoids. Women who have undergone several pregnancies, those expecting twins or those suffering from hydramnios (an excessive quantity of amniotic fluid) are particularly likely to develop varicose veins. If you are troubled with varicose veins, good support stockings are a necessity. But the stockings must be worn from the moment you get out of bed. If you wait to put them on until later in the day, your legs will already be swollen, and the support stockings will be ineffective.

There are several precautions you can take which will help to avoid varicose veins.

• Do not stand for long periods of time.

• Walk for half-an-hour every day. Walking encourages the circulation.

• Whenever you sit, be sure that your legs are elevated. Your feet should be higher than your pelvis. A pillow under the mattress at the bottom of your bed will also help.

• Never cross your legs when you are sitting (Illust 17) or sit with a child on your knee.

• Pay special attention to the exercises which help to relax your legs.

• Do not wear heels more than an inch and a half high.

• A tepid, rather than a hot bath will prevent the veins from dilating.

If varicose veins persist after delivery, your doctor may recommend treatment, but in most cases they will disappear within three months.

Note that it is especially important to maintain good posture while you are pregnant. If you do so, you will avoid or reduce the symptoms of many of the problems which are common during pregnancy. Most important, you will feel much better than if you "slouch".

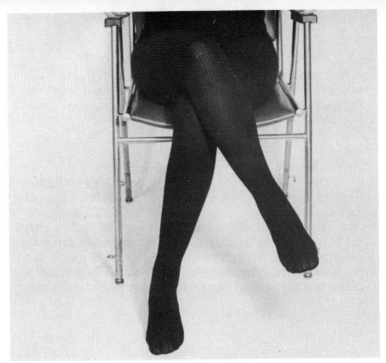

**Illust. 17**

As the uterus grows, you will begin to feel awkward, especially while walking. Contracting the muscles of the abdomen and buttocks straightens the spine and improves your posture. It also positions the uterus more comfortably and reduce the "bulge". (See Diagram 2) Always hold your shoulders up and try to keep your back straight when standing, walking or sitting. This keeps all your internal organs in their most comfortable positions and reduces the strain on the muscles of the abdomen and back.

**Hemorrhoids** This condition is common during pregnancy, and is an enlargement of the veins in the rectal area, similar to the varicose veins which may appear in the legs.

Avoid constipation. Eat lots of fresh fruit and green vegetables. Establish regular bowel movements and apply on ointment locally (your doctor will recommend one). Avoid hot baths.

**Stretch Marks** These are small, pinkish lines which may appear on the skin of the abdomen, upper thighs and sometimes on the breasts. They are caused by the stretching of the skin which ruptures some of the elastic fibres of the skin. These marks will not disappear completely, but after the birth of your baby, they will be less prominent and their colour will fade. To prevent or reduce stretch marks, it is a good idea to begin around the fourth month to massage a cream into the skin of the breasts and abdomen each day.

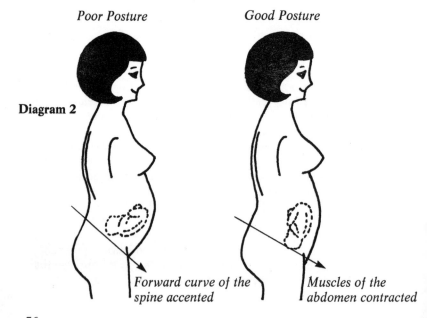

*Poor Posture*  *Good Posture*

**Diagram 2**

*Forward curve of the spine accented*

*Muscles of the abdomen contracted*

It is important to maintain the suppleness of the skin. Use a good quality cream with an oil base, or a good moisturizing lotion. There are several excellent anti-stretch mark creams available which are made especially for pregnant women. Also, be careful not to gain too much weight, since this can aggravate stretch marks.

**Diagram 3**

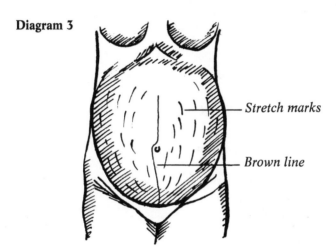

— *Stretch marks*

— *Brown line*

Around the 6th month your navel will become more prominent. This distention of the navel may occasionally cause a hernia.

**Edema**   Swelling of the ankles, legs, hands and/or face.

This is due to the accumulation or retention of water in the tissues. Tell your doctor who will test for the presence of albumin in the urine. If your blood pressure is too high and/or if you are having trouble with your vision, the doctor may prescribe a diuretic. In this case, you will urinate much more and will notice a loss of several pounds almost immediately.

**Toxemia of Pregnancy**   Poisoning of the system, leading to convulsions. This condition is quite rare today because more women are under the constant care of doctors throughout their pregnancies.

Symptoms of Toxemia

* rapid weight gain
* headaches
* swelling of hands, face and ankles
* distorted vision
* digestive upsets; nausea, vomiting, pains in the pit of the stomach
* decreased quantity of urine
* rise in blood pressure

# Symptoms of Serious Problems Requiring Immediate Attention

If any of the following symptoms appear, you should contact your doctor immediately.

* Pain when urinating, cloudy and/or foaming urine.

* Rapid weight gain. With a well-balanced diet you should gain from ½ to ¾ of a pound per week or from 3 pounds a month from the 3rd month on.

* Swelling of the feet, hands and face.

* Vision disorders: black spots in front of the eyes, or blurred vision.

* Persistant headaches which are not relieved by simple medication.

* Vaginal bleeding or spotting. This could be serious. Call your doctor and get into bed at once.

* Abdominal pains preceded by pains in the lumbar region. It is normal during the last stage of your pregnancy to feel these pains, commonly called false labour. They are due to the enlargement of the uterus and the movement of the fetus. (If the pains disappear after rest in bed or after a good night's sleep, they are probably caused by tension on the ligaments and muscles.)

* Absence of movement of the fetus for more than three days after the sixth month of pregnancy.

* Rupture of the membranes which is manifested by a loss of fluid through the vagina. Be sure that it is not a loss of urine. It is common during the final stages of pregnancy to have some difficulty controlling your bladder. This is caused by the heaviness of the uterus on the bladder.

* Decrease in the quantity of urine. You should urinate about 2 pints in each 24 hour period.

* Serious vomiting continuing after the fourth month.

* Repeated fainting.

## Should You Change Your Pattern of Living?

Pregnancy is no longer considered a delicate condition. There is no reason to curtail your activities to any great extent. Common sense is a good guide and excesses should be avoided. Especially during the first three months, get as much extra rest as possible and do not engage in violent sports or take tiring trips.

## Should You Continue to Work?

If you are working outside the home, there is no reason why you can't continue doing so until the 7th month. However, this too, should be tempered with common sense. Do not work overtime, or lift or carry heavy objects. Avoid standing for long periods. You will notice that towards the end of your pregnancy, your sense of balance will be affected. Be especially careful of falls at this time.

If you want to decorate the new baby's room, you can do the planning, but let your husband do the work.

## Should You Continue to Participate in Sports?

The type of sport in which you should engage during pregnancy depends largely upon what you are accustomed to. It is not, however, a good time to take up something new or to enter competitions.

There are certain sports that are not good, such as bicycling, motorcycling, horseback riding, skiing, skating, snowmobiling, tennis, badminton or any of the violent sports which have direct action on the muscles of the pelvis and abdomen. Such activities could cause a premature rupture of the membrane or a detachment of the placenta. The sports which are suitable are swimming (not diving), golf (9 holes will probably be enough for you), bowling if you are accustomed to it and walking half an hour in the fresh air every day. Walking activates the circulation, particularly in the legs, encourages the functioning of the intestine, reinforces the abdominal muscles, and helps position the fetus properly. You are advised, however, to reduce this half hour to a quarter hour during the ninth month.

### Prenatal Swimming (Illust. 18)

Swimming is a sport which every future mother can enjoy safely. It is an excellent way to relax and the breathing techniques used are complimentary to those you will learn in your prenatal classes.

You should be careful not to stretch your legs while swimming, since this may cause cramps in your legs. Of course you should not dive or over-exert yourself. As in all sports, common sense is your best guide. Swimming can be a very enjoyable experience, especially since the water supports your weight and you feel light and supple. (Illust. 18a)

**Illust. 18**

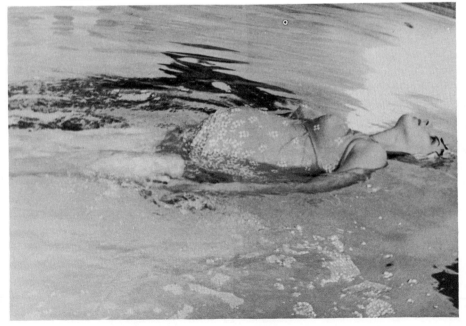

## Should You Stop Smoking?

Cigarettes, like alcohol, are not recommended for the pregnant woman. If you cannot stop smoking altogether, at least do not smoke more than 10 cigarettes a day. When tempted to take a cigarette, take five deep breaths instead. Smoking activates respiration, but the nicotine may be harmful to your fetus.

You will have more difficulty tolerating alcohol during pregnancy. Both liquor and wine may also produce heartburn.

## Should You Travel?

Air travel is not recommended during the first three months, and some airlines refuse to accept pregnant women after their 7th month because of the danger of premature delivery.

**Illust. 18a**

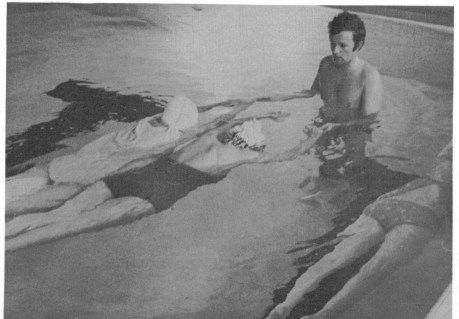

Long trips by car should be taken in easy stages, with stops every two hours. This will give you an opportunity to stretch your legs and visit the ladies' room. An asset on a long trip is a rubber cushion to protect you from the bumps. It is inadvisable to drive your car during the last weeks of pregnancy. Your reflexes are considerably slower and you are bound to be uncomfortable trying to squeeze behind the steering wheel.

Boat travel presents the hazard of seasickness (and if the trip is of long duration there is the added hazard of lack of medical facilities, should you need them.)

## Should You Take Baths?

You should take a bath every day during pregnancy, especially because you will perspire more as the body attempts to eliminate the increase of waste products. The only time when baths are forbidden is when there is any show of blood, or after the membranes have ruptured or when albumin is present in the urine.

Since vaginal secretions are more abundant during pregnancy, you should be especially careful to cleanse the genital area at least once each day. Baths also have a sedative effect and will help you to sleep better. Add a teaspoon of salt, bicarbonate of soda or a relaxing foam to your bath water.

Warm baths are preferable, since hot water dilates the blood vessels, thus encouraging the development of varicose veins. Cold baths, besides being uncomfortable, are unwise because they could start contractions. Sauna baths are definitely not recommended, since the perspiring can cause weakness and faintness.

Follow your bath with a brisk rub-down with a towel, then apply a good moisturizing body lotion to help maintain the suppleness of your skin.

Vaginal douches are forbidden without your doctor's advice.

## Should You Wear a Girdle?

A girdle simply does the work that the abdominal muscle should do. If you depend on a girdle, your muscles will lose their elasticity. Strong abdominal muscles will support the uterus well, and these muscles can be strengthened by doing your prenatal exercises every day after the third month.

Girdles are useful in certain pregnancies. Women whose muscles have been weakened by several pregnancies, or who are carrying twins may be advised by their doctors to wear one. Girdles are also recommended in the case of a navel hernia or when there is slackening of the ligaments which attach the bones of the pelvis.

## What is a "Pregnancy Mask"?

Some women — not many — may notice a darkish discolouration of the skin over the cheeks, on the upper lip or on each side of the chin. If this should occur, avoid exposure to the sun without a protective cream. This is another condition which will disappear after the birth of the baby.

### Skin Care

You should pay special attention to your skin and makeup during pregnancy. Makeup should be carefully removed from face and neck each night. Use any good cleansing agent which is appropriate for your type of skin. A moisturizing cream should be used overnight. If your skin is dry, apply a moisturizing lotion before your makeup during the day. A reputable beautician will be happy to advise you on the choice and use of these products.

Learn the art of applying eye makeup skillfully. (Putting your eyes in the spotlight is a clever way of diverting attention from your new figure) A visit to the hairdresser is as good for the appearance as it is for the morale.

Emotional ups and downs are a natural part of pregnancy. A glance at your silhouette in the mirror can easily spark a fit of the "blues". When this happens, a trip to the hairdresser is an excellent investment and is as good for the morale as it is for the appearance. In addition to the other cosmetic aids you may use, be sure that you have a good cleansing cream, a daytime and nightime cream, a cream to prevent stretch marks and a moisturizing body lotion.

## Should You Wear a Bra?

Modern liberated women may be burning their bras, but if you are pregnant, wait until after your baby has been born.

The pectoral muscles support the mammary glands (breasts) and, as your breasts grow heavy, the muscles may become stretched. It is, therefore, necessary to wear a good supportive bra. In Chapter V there are exercises to strengthen the pectoral muscles.

The breasts may increase in weight from 2 to 3 pounds during pregnancy. They also, of course, increase in size and your bra size may change several times. Be sure to change the size when required. A bra that is too tight is not only uncomfortable, but could be harmful. There are special maternity bras available which provide the necessary support. Some women wear a bra day and night during the last month, and for the first few weeks after delivery. This is a matter of personal comfort.

It is quite normal for a network of blue veins to appear on the breasts. These will disappear after delivery. You will also notice a whitish discharge from the nipple. This fluid is called *colostrum* and is the first sign that milk is forming in your breasts. Wash the nipples carefully with clear warm water and rinse with cool water. This will prevent the colostrum from hardening around the nipple and help to keep the skin from cracking.

## What is a Caesarian Section?

A Caesarian section is the surgical removal of the fetus from the mother's womb. The decision to perform a Caesarian section is made by your doctor after careful consideration of your condition and any special problems you may have. Caesarians are performed only when absolutely necessary, that is, when the life of the child or the mother is endangered, or when the mother is physically unable to stand the strain of a normal delivery. For example, if the mother has serious respiratory problems, a heart or kidney condition, or if she suffers from diabetis, the doctor will consider a Caesarian. In cases where the mother has a congenital malformation of the uretus, or *dystonia* of the uterus (incapacity of tissue to stretch), a Caesarian is usually indicated. If the fetus is endangered in any way, or if there are obvious signs of fetal exertion like a change in the sound of the heart or stained amniotic fluid, the doctor will consider this method of delivery. In any case, a Caesarian section is a major surgical procedure and is never undertaken without sound medical reasons.

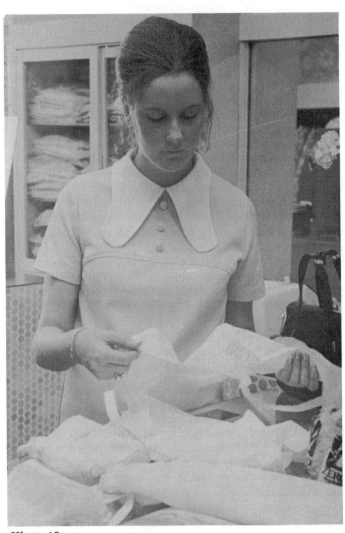

**Illust. 19**

## What About Your Sex Life?

It is a good idea to ref ain from sexual activity during the last month of pregnanc order to avoid the risk of infection or premature rupture of the membrane. From a purely practical standpoint, a woman in the last month of pregnancy may find sexual intercourse an awkward activity.

## Should You Nurse your Baby?

The pros and cons of breast feeding have been argued for generations. Today it is more in vogue than it was in our mothers' day. Discuss the subject with your doctor and, if possible, with a friend who has breast fed her own baby. Try to find as much factual information as possible, but do not listen to the old wives' tales which abound in this subject. In many cities and communities there are groups of young mothers who meet regularly to discuss breast feeding and who will be happy to answer your questions and help you build your confidence. Your doctor or the hospital may be able to locate such a group in your community. Certainly, you should be well informed on the subject before you make a final decision. There are, of course, several excellent books available, and you will no doubt want to read at least one of these. Again, ask your doctor for his recommendation.

If you do decide to breast feed your child, ask your doctor to arrange with the nursery in the hospital to bring the child to you every 3 hours instead of every 4 as is the custom in most hospitals. More frequent feedings will ensure that you always have enough milk, because the child will take less at each feeding, as he will be less hungry. You may have some discomfort in your breasts when you first begin to nurse, but this will not last long.

In some hospitals, the baby is kept in the mother's room during the day, and she cares for him herself. Of course the baby is removed to the nursery at night so the mother can sleep. This is an excellent practice, especially for mothers having their first child. When they are ready to go home, they are accustomed to caring for the child and are not nervous when handling him.

If you are nursing your baby, remember that you must get lots of rest in order to ensure a sufficient supply of milk. Also, you must visit your doctor once a month for at least 6 months, and have regular check-up after that for as long as you continue to nurse.

New mothers frequently experience a period of depression which contrasts sharply with the feeling of euphoria and happiness which immediately follows the birth. Two or three days after delivery it is not uncommon for young mothers to dissolve in tears and express worries and doubts about the child and their ability to feed it. This is a quite natural emotional reaction to the sudden physical changes which have just taken place in your body. It will pass in a few days.

# The Do's and Don'ts of Pregnancy

## Do's

- Get 8 — 10 hours of sleep a night
- Nap in the afternoon if possible
- Walk half an hour every day
- Do breathing and physical exercises which you will learn in your prenatal classes
- Wear a good bra
- Bathe every day
- Maintain a sensible diet
- Take the vitamins and any other medication prescribed by your doctor
- Maintain good posture
- Visit your doctor regularly

**Don'ts**

- Do not smoke, or at least cut down to 10 or fewer cigarettes per day
- Avoid violent sports
- Avoid getting overtired
- Try not to have repeated late nights
- Stay out of draughts and do not catch cold
- Cut down on salt, especially after the 4th month
- Do not overeat
- Avoid an excessive weight gain
- Avoid long trips
- Do not listen to gossip or old wives' tales about childbirth
- Avoid contact with people (especially young children) who have contagious diseases

# Chapter III

## Some Practical Advice

There are several positions which are especially comfortable and beneficial and which can be used when you are doing housework or just relaxing.

### The "Tailor" Position (Illust. 20)

You should become accustomed to doing many small daily jobs in this position. You can mend, knit, read, watch television, and even do some kitchen work like preparing vegetables while seated comfortably in this position which is similar to the lotus position in yoga. A child takes this position quite naturally. Watch him while he is looking at his picture books or his favourite television program. While it is ideal for preparing the muscles for delivery, it is not the most elegant position and probably should not be assumed in the living room when you have guests!

The "tailor" position has several important advantages:

— It pushes the uterus forward, where it belongs and is most comfortable.

— The muscles on the inside of the thighs stretch and become supple.

— The groin region is strengthened, thus facilitating delivery because the muscles are supple and stretch easily.

— It strengthens the muscles which support the bladder and uterus, thus eliminating many cases of *prolapse* (falling) of these organs.

— It helps to prevent varicose veins and hemorroids.

Note, however, that this position should not be taken for long periods, especially by older women who are not accustomed to it. You will feel a pulling sensation in your groin and on the inner thighs. This is due to a lack of suppleness in the joints and will disappear with time, as the joints become more supple.

To relax from the "tailor" position, stretch your legs out and slap the calf of each leg vigourously against the floor.

When sitting in a chair, it is not a good idea to let yourself slide down into a slouching position with your spine bent. This causes the uterus to drop deeply into the pelvis instead of falling freely forward. In addition, the blood vessels which irrigate the kidneys and the legs are compressed and the circulation is restricted. Also, slouching encourages the appearance of the "dowager's hump" and thus tires the neck and shoulders.

## The Squatting Position (Illust. 21)

You have many opportunities during the day to use the squatting position which exercises the muscles of the back, stomach and perineum.

**Illust. 20**

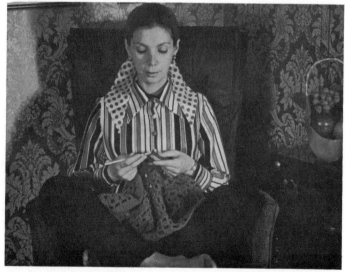

A woman who has no children can bend over twenty times in the course of a day — to pick up an object, dust, put utensils into low cupboards, lift a pet, or in gardening and many other tasks both in the house and outside. A mother with small children can bend over up to a hundred times a day! Make use of all these opportunities to strengthen your muscles by squatting rather than bending from the waist.

As your pregnancy advances, you will find bending difficult — it will be uncomfortable and you will feel short of breath.

**Illust. 21**

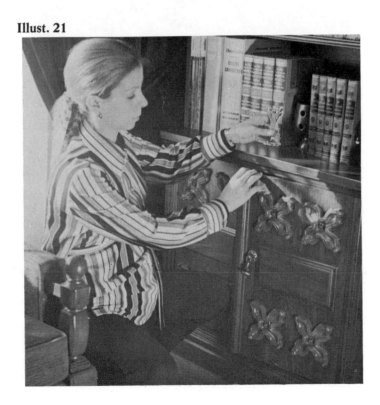

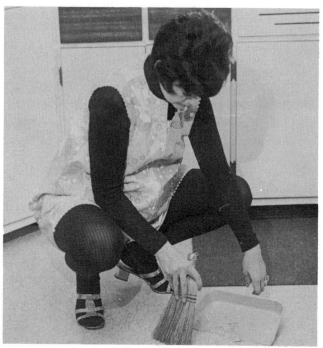

**Illust. 22**

Instead, spread your knees and squat with your back straight (Illust. 22) This position helps to soften the perineum and this will shorten the period of labour before delivery. Squatting also reinforces the abdominal wall and the dorsal muscles. The squatting position can decrease the possibility of "breech" birth. The incidence of breech birth among primitive people is rare.

## The Seated Position (Illust. 23)

Learn to do much of your housework while sitting down. Get a high stool with a back, making sure it is comfortable, with a rung for your feet. You can do many kitchen tasks while seated, like baking, washing dishes, planning meals,

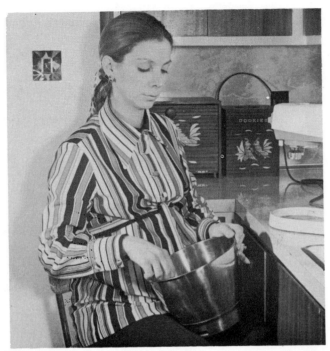

**Illust. 23**

etc. Your circulation will be improved and you will be less subject to varicose veins and heaviness in your legs. Always sit well back and keep your shoulders straight — this will help to eliminate back ache.

The high stool is especially useful for ironing since standing to iron encourages a curve in the back. (Illust. 24) Lower your ironing board to the correct height and sit on the stool. (Illust. 25) You will find that you do not become tired so quickly, and that your legs do not ache.

A familiar movement, made several times a day, is that of bending to place an object on the ground or to lift a basket of clothes or a child or a pet. Bending from the waist with

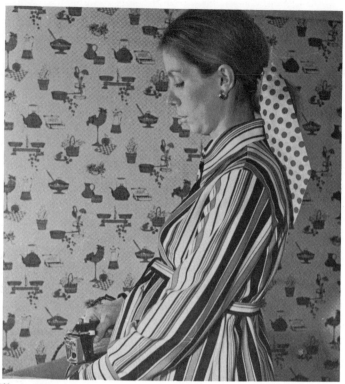

**Illust. 24**

stiff knees is both uncomfortable and ungraceful. (Illust. 27)
Instead, train yourself to bend your legs, knees separated,
keeping your back straight. (Illust. 26) The lifting is supplied
by the arms and legs, not by the muscles of the back and
stomach. Remember that you should never bend your back
when you can bend your legs.

Lifting an object with outstretched arms can cause severe
back pain, because the back must curve forward sharply.
(Illust. 28)

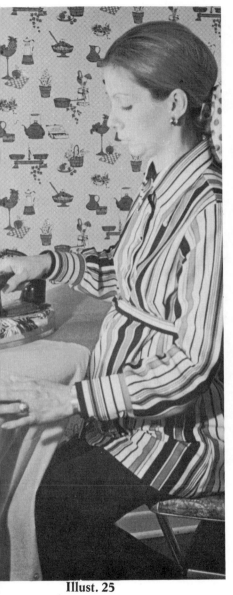

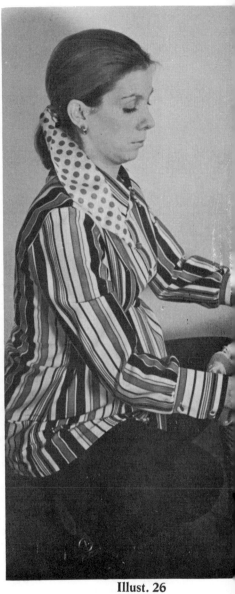

Illust. 25                              Illust. 26

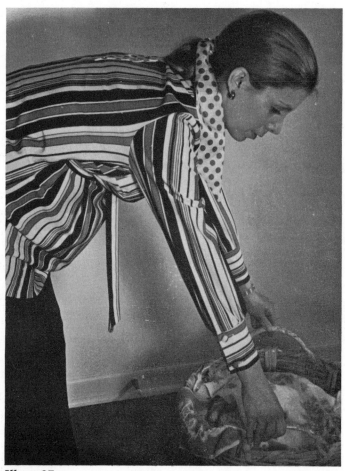

**Illust. 27**

Instead, bend your knees, keep your back straight and contract the abdominal muscles. (Illust. 29) Even if the object to be lifted is heavy, you will not feel the pull of the ligaments in your back.

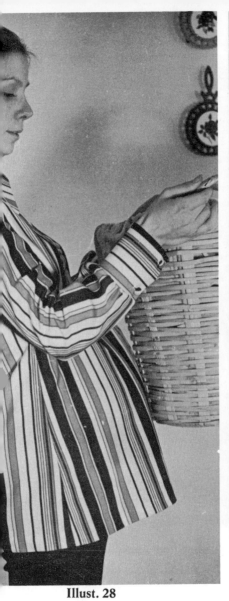

Illust. 28

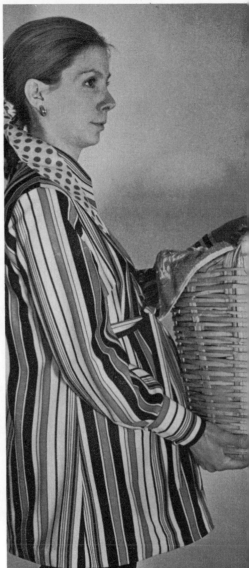

Illust. 29

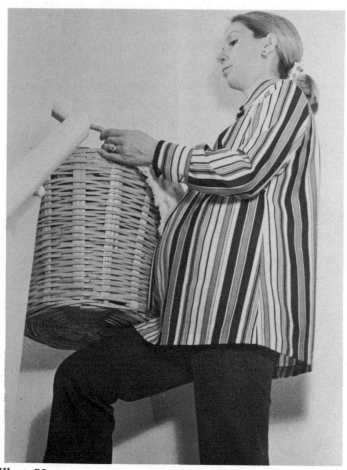

**Illust. 30**

If your laundry room is in the basement and it is necessary to make several trips up and down stairs carrying a laundry basket, you should take care not to climb the stairs too quickly. Walk up four steps and stop, resting the basket on one knee, (Illust. 30) then walk up four more steps and rest again, until you reach the top. Breathe deeply while climbing and try not to carry too heavy loads in your laundry

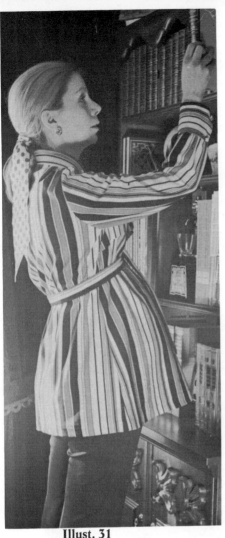 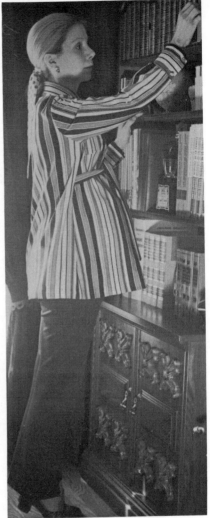

| Illust. 31 | Illust. 32 |
|---|---|

basket. If you become tired, stop work and lie down with your feet elevated for a few minutes until you feel rested.

To reach an object on a high shelf, you must stretch properly. Do not bend your back (lean backward) in order to raise your arms. (Illust. 31) Instead, contract your abdominal muscles and stand on tiptoe as you raise your arms. (Illust. 32) Do not stand on a chair or other piece of furniture to

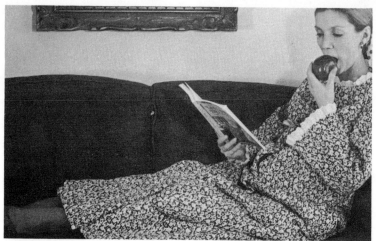

Illust. 33

Illust. 34

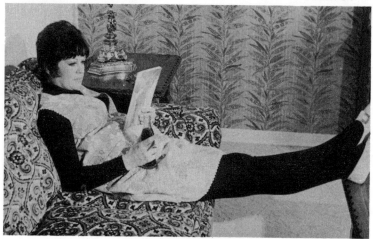

reach an object on a very high shelf. Wait until your
husband can get it for you. It is very easy to lose your
balance when you look down.

Take some time in the afternoon for a rest. Encourage circulation by raising your legs to the same height as the pelvis
or higher. (Illust. 33) Eating fruit as a snack is much better

than drinking a soft drink and eating potato chips or smoking a cigarette. (Illust. 34)

You should pay particular attention to your posture while you are pregnant. Poor posture slackens the abdominal muscles and frequently causes back ache.

### Some Helpful Hints

• To get out of bed easily, lie on your side, (Illust. 35), then raise your trunk by means of your lower arm and lower your feet off the bed. (Illust. 36)

• Never stretch your legs and feet during pregnancy. This can cause cramps in the calves and feet.

• Sitting down gracefully can be a very effective exercise for the back muscles. Do not let yourself fall into a chair, but

**Illust. 35**

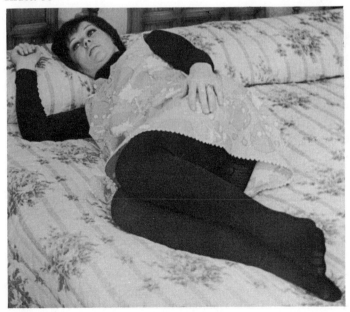

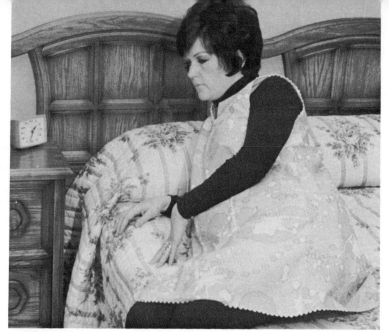

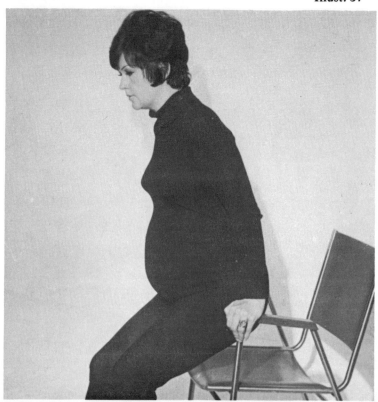

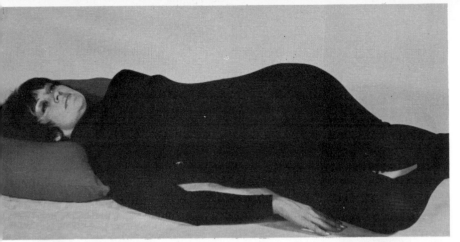

Illust. 38                                                    Illust. 39

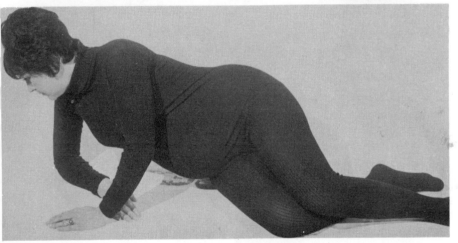

keep your balance by making your leg muscles work. (Illust. 37) The same principle applies for getting up again. Slide to the edge of the chair and contract your leg muscles.

You will probably do your daily exercises on the floor. When you have finished, rest briefly on your back with one knee bent.

To get up, roll onto your right side. (Illust. 38) Raise your shoulders with the help of your lower right arm and your left hand. (Illust. 39) Sit with your knees bent, hands on

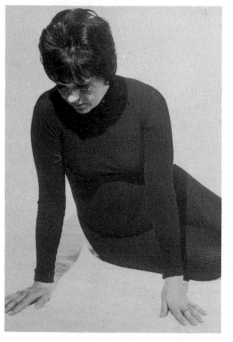

**Illust. 40**

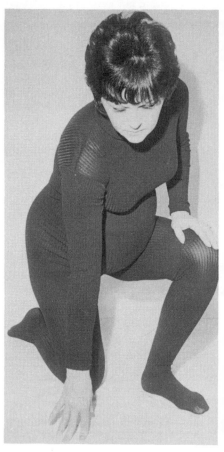

**Illust. 41**

the floor, resting briefly. (Illust. 40) Then continue the movement by leaving the right knee on the floor and placing the left hand on the left knee. (Illust. 41)

# Sensible Eating

The legend that you should "eat for two" when you are pregnant is quite without foundation in fact. If you eat twice as much, you will gain far too much weight and will be overweight after your baby is born. You must, of course, maintain a healthy diet. Your health before and after delivery depends on your diet and the health of your baby depends on the quality of the food you eat. Planning your menus can be an enjoyable task, and is best left to your own taste and imagination. However, there are certain foods which should be included in your diet, and others which should be avoided.

**Proteins** are necessary to build and repair tissues. Good sources of protein are red and white meats, poultry, fish, eggs, dairy products and cereals.

**Vitamins** are necessary to ensure good health for both you and your baby. Vitamin A is found in milk, eggs, butter, margarine and vegetables such as beans, broccoli, asparagus, spinach and carrots. It promotes growth and aids development of the eyes.

Vitamin B is found in milk, meat (especially liver), whole wheat cereals and eggs, and is used mainly in the development and maintenance of the nervous system.

Vitamin C is found in citrus fruits like oranges, grapefruit and lemons, and in tomatoes, apple juice and cabbage. It helps to prevent infections, colds and flu.

Vitamin D is not provided in sufficient quantities in the foods we eat to supply the needs of a pregnant woman. It is necessary for the assimilation of calcium which is indispensible to the formation of bones and teeth. In order to have enough Vitamin D to maintain your own bones and teeth and to build strong bones and teeth in your baby, you must take Vitamin D in tablet form.

The sun is an excellent source of Vitamin D, and if you are pregnant during the summer you can enjoy moderate sunbathing.

## Fats and Sugars

A normal, balanced diet provides sufficient quantities of fats and sugars. In fact, many diets contain too much bread, cake, candy, rich sauce, etc. Any of these foods eaten in large quantities will add to your weight.

### Some Hints

• Eat several small meals a day rather than three large meals. You will feel more comfortable and digest your food more easily.

• Eat 100% whole wheat bread rather than white bread. Eat bread only at one meal, in the morning, for example, in the form of toast.

• Eat eggs at least two or three times a week, or more often if you like. Fried eggs with bacon are not recommended, since bacon contains too much salt and fried foods may cause heartburn. Instead, boil or poach your eggs.

• One portion of meat each day is sufficient, preferably broiled.

• Eat fish at least three times a week, preferably poached or baked.

• Eat cooked vegetables, but also at least one raw vegetable daily, preferably a salad with either vegetable oil, lemon or yogurt dressing. Get into the habit of keeping carrot sticks, celery, radishes or pieces of cucumber, in the refrigerator for between-meal snacks. (Illust. 42)

Drink at least two large glasses of milk each day. Eat all the yogurt and cottage cheese you want. Milk-based desserts such as custard and puddings are especially good.

Eat lots of fresh fruit — oranges, grapefruits, apples, and bananas — and use fresh lemon juice in salads and cooking. Fruit is no more expensive than rich desserts, and is much better for you.

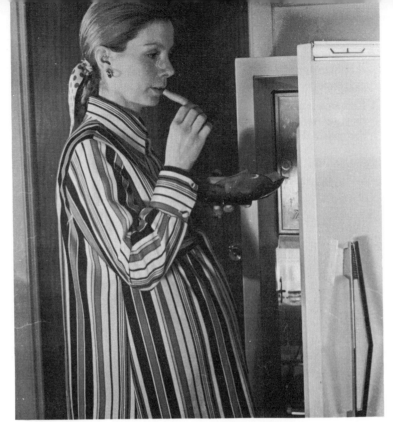

**Illust. 42**

Use as little white sugar as possible. Instead, use natural brown unrefined sugar.

Drink lots of freshly squeezed vegetable juice between meals or before your meals.

Avoid soft drinks and spicy foods, such as Chinese food, pizza and spaghetti. Cut down on (or eliminate from your diet entirely) cakes, doughnuts, pies and whipped cream.

Do not use salt on your food after the fourth month of pregnancy. You may use salt when cooking vegetables.

The elimination of salt during the last four months encourages the functioning of the uterine muscle and reduces the resistance of the striated muscles of the perineum during delivery.

Remember that a well-balanced diet is essential to the health of your baby. Remember, too, that the less weight you gain, the easier the delivery will be.

# Chapter IV

## Physical and Psychological Preparation for Pregnancy

One of the myths still surrounding pregnancy is the inevitable effect it will have on a woman's appearance. Many women think they will never again be attractive. They picture themselves going through life overweight and out of shape. Of course, this can happen if no precautions are taken. A woman who eats exactly what she pleases and never exercises will have a difficult time regaining her slim figure.

There was a time when pregnancy was considered an illness and, at least for the affluent woman, meant almost total inactivity. She spent her days confined to bed, at least lounging on a sofa. She remained almost totally inactive, avoiding exercise and baths because both were considered to be dangerous to the fetus.

On the other hand, a peasant woman simply ignored pregnancy. She continued to work in the fields, "ate for two", and, if she availed herself of the services of a doctor, it was only when her labour pains began. She resigned herself to a lifetime of pregnancies. Her condition was never discussed with her friends, it was considered almost shameful.

Today, the outlook is quite different. A couple can now plan their family and "surprise" pregnancies are relatively rare. Thus, the future mother accepts her pregnancy with serenity and joy and is anxious to tell her friends and relatives the good news. She consults a doctor from the very beginning and learns all she can about the life developing within her body. She attends prenatal classes and learns how to care for herself during pregnancy.

Most importantly, she is conscious of the creative aspect of her role and eagerly shares her knowledge with her husband.

## Conditioning Exercises for Childbirth

The importance of exercise during your pregnancy cannot be overemphasized. Mild exercise promotes a feeling of well-being and comfort, and improves circulation and breathing. Exercise also encourages good posture, which, in turn, will prevent backache and promote good digestion.

If your muscles have been firmed through exercise and your joints are supple, the length of labour will be reduced and your figure will return to normal more rapidly after the birth of your child.

All of the exercises in this book have been especially designed for pregnant women and are neither strenuous nor complicated. They are exercises which would normally be included in prenatal classes, whether conducted in a hospital or private clinic. Each exercise is clearly illustrated and described. Your husband can play a very important role in encouraging you to do your exercises and in helping you over the "rough spots" when you become discouraged.

## The Prenatal Class

The purpose of a prenatal class is to help you to learn to relax and breathe properly so that you will be prepared for the delivery of your child. Psychological preparation for childbirth is also an important part of the prenatal class — and cannot easily be accomplished on your own. The help and encouragement you will receive from a competent instructor will be invaluable to you. You will be enormously pleased to discover how supple you can be and how much better you will feel as you perform the rhythm exercises which make up part of your prenatal classes.

If you are accustomed to engaging in active sports, such as horseback riding or bicycling, you will find that your prenatal exercises may not take the place of these activities, but they do allow you some moderate physical activity.

With your doctor's permission, you may begin exercising around the fourth month. Some doctors prefer to wait until the first movements of the fetus are felt — this usually occurs around the fourth or fifth month. Even if you wait to begin exercising until your pregnancy is further advanced, the results will still be beneficial to you.

Choose a quiet, well-ventilated room to do your exercises. Place a rug, towel or mat on the floor — a mattress is not recommended. Have two pillows available.

Wear a bra that fits properly, but do not wear a girdle. It is impossible to contract your abdominal muscles properly while wearing a girdle. Wear a gym suit or tights and a maternity top. It is preferable to be barefoot.

Twenty minutes of combined physical and breathing exercises is sufficient. Relax completely between exercises in order to prevent fatigue. After finishing your exercises, remain on the floor, completely relaxed, for about ten minutes. Try to make your mind a blank during this time.

Avoid stretching both legs at the same time; this could cause backache. Do not point your toes; this could cause leg cramps.

Never get up quickly after lying on your back. Turn over on your side and push yourself up with your hands. (See Illust. 38-41)

Especially during a first pregnancy, it is a great advantage to attend a prenatal clinic, rather than to exercise at home alone. Without supervision, it is easy to do an exercise incorrectly. If you are on your own, you may start off with great enthusiasm and continue for a few weeks, but the temptation to slow down will be strong. Working with a group is far more interesting and stimulating. The very fact that you must get out of the house in order to attend a class is good for you in that you will make an effort to improve your appearance. One of the most important assets of the prenatal class is the fellowship that you will encounter in a group.

On your own, there is a tendency to magnify your problems; when you meet regularly with others who share the same condition, you gain perspective and your problems no longer seem so important.

Women who have attended prenatal classes during the course of other pregnancies will recognize the advantages of these classes. They will also find this book a valuable aid in helping them recall what they have already learned. If you are unable to attend prenatal classes, or if you live in an area where prenatal classes are not available, this book, along with the encouragement of your doctor, will help you to prepare for this all-important event.

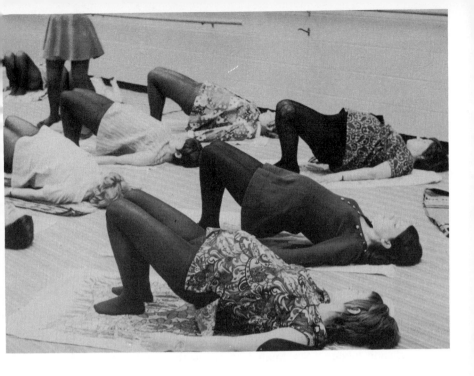

## Relaxation

With all the strains and pressures of modern living, the ability to relax is an important step towards mental and physical health. Most people who have not been trained in the art of relaxation have no idea how to achieve it. When *required* to relax, the natural tendency is to contract the muscles, thus achieving the opposite effect. It is especially important for you to know how to relax when you are pregnant and careful attention to these exercises will certainly help you to be more relaxed. Remember that tension builds up daily and so must be relieved daily. It is not sufficient to do relaxation exercises once a week, they must be done each day.

You must train yourself to relax when you want to. Do not assume that relaxation is simply stretching out on a sofa, chair or rug and letting your muscles go limp. Physical relaxation cannot be separated from mental relaxation. If your mind is filled with worries and problems you will not be able to relax properly. Concentrate on a peaceful scene, a beautiful painting, or perhaps the face of someone you love. You will immediately feel a sense of peace. This, combined with relaxed muscles, is real relaxation.

Every pregnant woman requires, even searches for a feeling of calmness and peace. The noise and discord of radio, television, even household appliances will become more and more troublesome to you while you are pregnant. The relaxation which can be achieved by doing these exercises will be important to your sense of serenity. Try not to let outside influences bother you — emotional stress should be avoided if at all possible.

The effort made to learn to relax will be well rewarded during labour. A woman who is unable to relax at will is very likely to automatically contract her muscles when she feels the onset of a labour pain. This, of course, is the worst thing she can do and simply increases the pain.

To relieve pain, the proper procedure is to relax your muscles as you have learned to do, breathing deeply at the same time.

The importance of learning this skill is obvious when you contrast what happens during labour to two women, one who has mastered the technique and one who has not.

A woman who is properly prepared for childbirth is happy about her condition because she understands it and her role in the delivery of her child. She knows the physiology of pregnancy and the process of childbirth. She is calm and serene and knows how to relax. Because of this, she is able to breathe properly and control her contractions. She understands that each contraction helps to achieve the dilation of the neck of the womb, thus bringing her closer to the moment of delivery.

Childbirth is, for her, a positive experience, one of the most important of her life, which she may well be able to share with her husband. She is able to co-operate fully at the moment of delivery and to hear her child's first cry with a feeling of joy and excitement.

(Some hospitals allow your husband to be present for the delivery. His sharing of this all-important event will create a permanent bond within the family.)

On the other hand, a woman who is not properly prepared for childbirth is unable to relax. She does not fully understand what is happening and is therefore nervous and afraid. Because of her fear, she will be tense and will experience some pain, she will feel hostility toward the baby, perhaps even to the extent of saying she does not want the child.

The unprepared mother will dread each contraction and has no desire to be conscious at the moment of delivery. Her husband will not be allowed in the delivery room, and this will cause her to feel abandoned. She will remember her child's birth with bitterness.

## Exercises for Total Relaxation

**Starting position**   Lie d  n on a firm surface, with a pillow under your head and c   or two pillows under your thighs, so that your knees are a the same height as your stomach. (Illust. 43)

### First Exercise (Illust. 44)

Raise your arms, keeping your elbows straight. With arms extended, form a fist with each hand. Contract your arm and shoulder muscles as much as possible. Inhale slowly. Relax your muscles while exhaling slowly.

### Second Exercise (Illust. 45)

Hold your arms at your sides, slightly away from the body. Relax the muscles of your arms completely, thumb and index finger touching to form a circle.

Raise both legs twelve inches off the ground while inhaling. Contract the thigh muscles. (Remember not to point your toes.) Lower your legs slowly, exhaling as you do so.

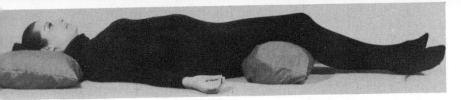

**Illust. 43**

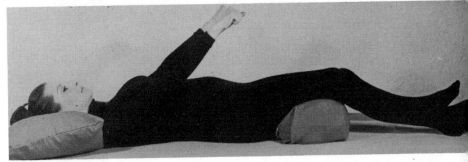

**Illust. 44**

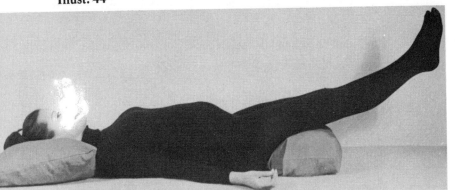

**Illust. 45**

### Third Exercise (Illust. 46)

Tighten the muscles of the left arm and right leg, allowing the muscles of the right arm and left leg to relax.

Tighten the muscles of the left arm and right leg, allowing the muscles of the left arm and right leg to relax.

### Fourth Exercise (Illust. 47)

Tighten the muscles of the left leg only, allowing the right leg and both arms to remain relaxed.

Tighten the muscles of the right leg, allowing the left leg and both arms to remain relaxed.

Raise your right arm in front of you, make a fist and tighten the muscles, allowing the left arm and both legs to remain relaxed.

Raise your left arm in front of you, make a fist and tighten the muscles, allowing the right arm and both legs to remain relaxed.

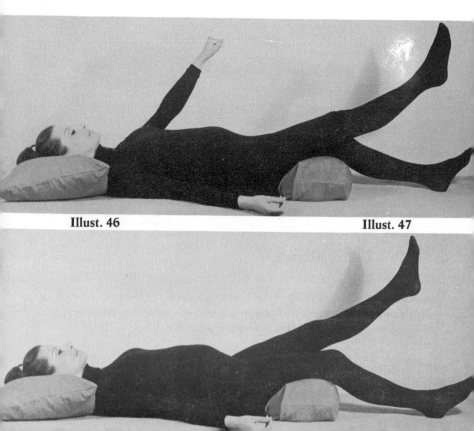

**Illust. 46**　　　　　　　　　　　　　**Illust. 47**

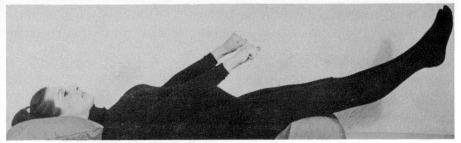

Illust. 48

Illust. 49

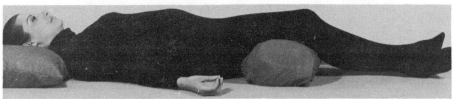

### Fifth Exercise (Illust. 48)

Raise both arms and both legs as far as possible from the floor. Then lower them slowly and relax the whole body.

## Comfortable Positions for Relaxation

• Lie on your back, one pillow under your head, two under your thighs. (Illust. 49)

This position is ideal for napping during the day as well as for relaxing between prenatal exercises. It is also a good position for sleeping during the first three months of pregnancy, since the uterus is not yet heavy enough to cause back pain. However, it is not recommended for sleeping during the last three months. It could interfere with the functioning of the kidneys and the circulation of blood to your legs. It could also cause backache.

Note that the pillows under your legs should be under your **thighs**, not in the hollow of your knees where the pressure might cut off circulation and thus promote varicose veins.

• Lie on your side, with three-quarters of your body resting on the abdomen. (Illust. 50)

Do not be afraid of harming the baby in this position. The fetus is well protected by the amniotic fluid. It is a good position for sleeping until the fifth or sixth month, when the size of the uterus becomes too large for this position to be comfortable.

• Lie on your side with your legs drawn up, with or without a pillow under your thighs. (Illust. 51) This is an ideal position for sleeping, preferably on your right side.

• Lie on your right side with your legs drawn up, the left leg higher than the right. A pillow may be placed under the left thigh

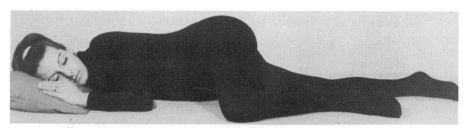

**Illust. 50**

**Illust. 51**

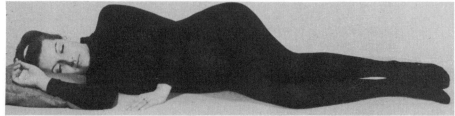

This position will ease tension on the sacro-uterine ligaments and allows the uterus to fall freely into the abdomen. It also improves circulation and will reduce swelling in the ankles.

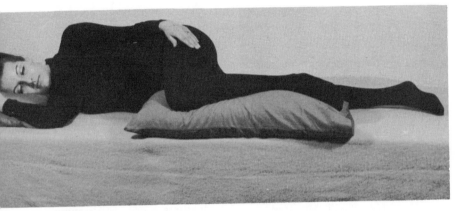

**Illust. 52**

## Breathing

Proper breathing aids digestion and helps you to relax and sleep — all important factors in pregnancy. The fetus needs oxygen in order to develop and the pregnant woman should appreciate the role she plays in supplying her baby with oxygen. A conscious effort must be made to breathe properly and in order to do so it is important to understand what takes place in the lungs and chest cavity during breathing.

### Respiration has two phases (Diagram 4)

**First phase** This is the inhaling or active phase. The lungs fill with oxygen, the pulmonary alveolae unfold (like a dry sponge when placed in water). The intercostal muscles separate, the diaphragm lowers, the chest cavity enlarges.

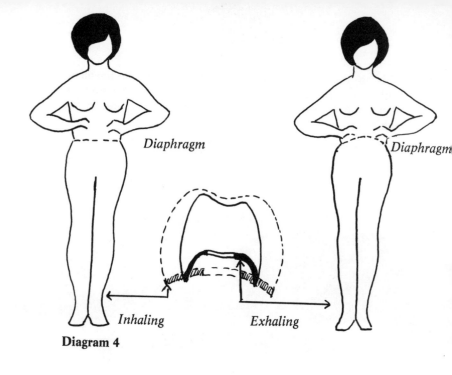

Diaphragm

Diaphragm

Inhaling          Exhaling

**Diagram 4**

**Second phase** This is the exhaling or passive phase. Carbon dioxide is released through the mouth. The lungs empty. The chest cavity contracts. The diaphragm rises and resumes its original position.

Note that the diaphragm is the smooth, dome-shaped muscle which separates the chest cavity from the abdominal cavity.

## Breathing Exercises

### Chest Breathing (Illust. 53)

Stand, legs together, place your two hands under your breasts on the rib-cage fingers touching.

a) Fill your lungs with air, inhaling through the nose to the count of four — the rib-cage will expend. Do not raise your shoulders while inhaling.

b) Exhale very slowly through your mouth, while counting six.

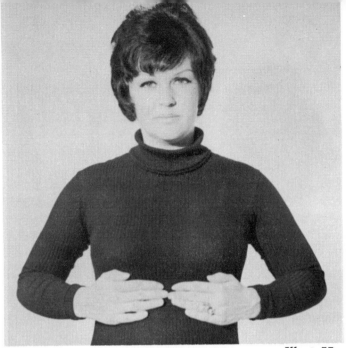

**Illust. 53**

### Chest Breathing (Illust. 54)

Lie on your back with a pillow under your head, your hands under your breasts on the rib-cage, fingers touching. Inhale through the nose to the count of six, filling your lungs with air, hold your breath to the count of ten and then exhale, mouth slightly open, to the count of eight.

### Chest Breathing (Illust. 55a and 55b)

Sit on the edge of a chair, feet together. Lift your arms at the sides to shoulder height.

a) Inhale through the nose, filling the lungs with air.

b) Let your arms fall slowly, dropping your arms to your sides in front of you and exhaling through the mouth. Relax the muscles of the back.

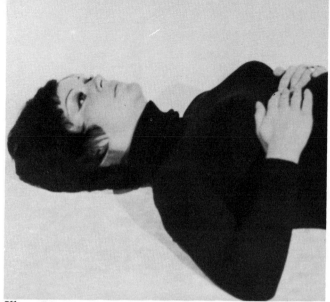

**Illust. 54**

### Abdominal Breathing (Illust. 56)

Deep abdominal breathing will help you during labour and also strengthens the abdominal wall. Lie on the floor, knees bent, feet on the floor, two hands on your abdomen.

a) Inhale through the nose to the count of four, pushing the abdomen out.

b) Exhale through the mouth to the count of six, while contracting the abdominal muscles.

### Complete Respiration

Lie on your back, knees bent, feet on the floor, a pillow under your head.

a) Inhale slowly through the nose, concentrating on the expansion of the rib-cage and abdomen and the flattening of the diaphragm.

b) Exhale slowly, the mouth half open.

Repeat six times.

Stand with your hands on your abdomen. (Illust. 57)

a) Inhale deeply through the nose. Feel your lungs fill with air and your abdomen expand.

b) Exhale with your mouth slightly open and feel the abdomen shrink.

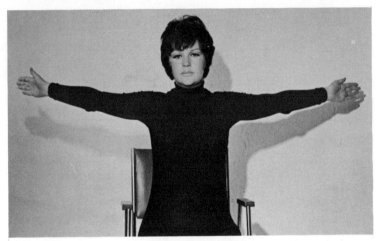

**Illust. 55a**

**Illust. 55b**

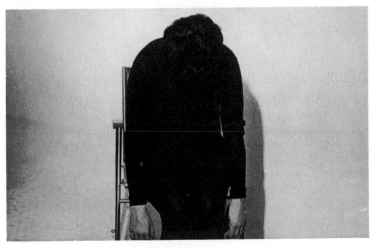

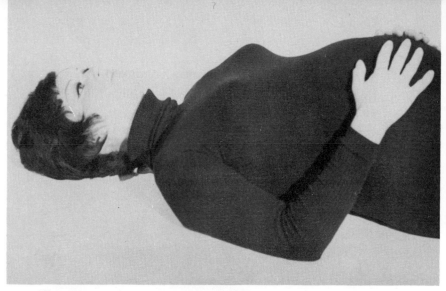

**Illust. 56**

**Illust. 57**

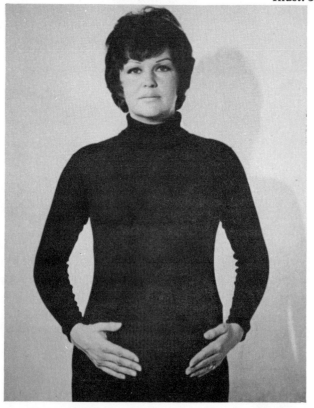

**Illust. 57**

# Chapter V

## Prenatal Exercises

Although the exercises described in this book are not strenuous, a twenty minute period of repetitious movement performed without interruption is too tiring and will produce muscular pain the following day unless precautions are taken. Proper breathing during each exercise will provide a certain amount of oxygen to the working muscles and will prevent stiffness. If one of the relaxation positions is assumed between each exercise, you will experience less fatigue. After each exercise period, take a warm bath to loosen your muscles and encourage relaxation.

## Exercises Designed to Promote Suppleness

### Exercise 1 (Illust. 58a and 58b)

Strengthens the anal area and softens the perineal muscles.

**Starting position** Sit on the floor "tailor" fashion with your back straight hands on your knees.

a) Inhale.

b) Lean forward, press your elbows against your knees, arch your back and let your head drop forward while exhaling.

Repeat four times if you are a beginner, eight times when you become accustomed to it.

### Exercise 2 (Illust. 59)

Eliminates tension in the groin and promotes suppleness in the perineum.

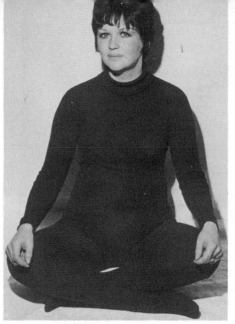 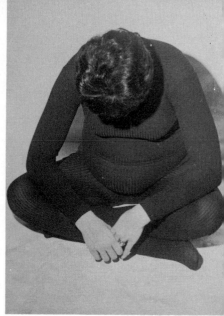

**Illust. 58a**                    **Illust. 58b**

**Starting position**  Sit on the floor, knees bent, soles of feet together. Grasp your feet in your hands and move your knees rapidly up and down.

Four times for beginners, eight for others.

### Exercise 3 (Illust. 60)

Strengthens the abdominal muscles.

**Starting position**  Lie on your back, a pillow under your head, right leg stretched out, left knee bent, arms at your sides.

a) Contract abdominal muscles, pressing the lumbar region against the floor, contracting the muscles as if trying to shorten your leg. Inhale.

b) Stretch out your right leg while exhaling.

c) Change legs and repeat.

Four times for beginners, eight for others.

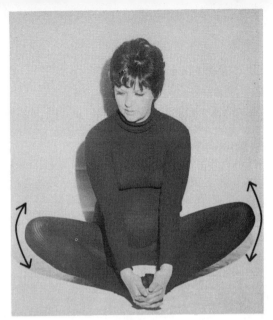

Illust. 59

Illust. 60

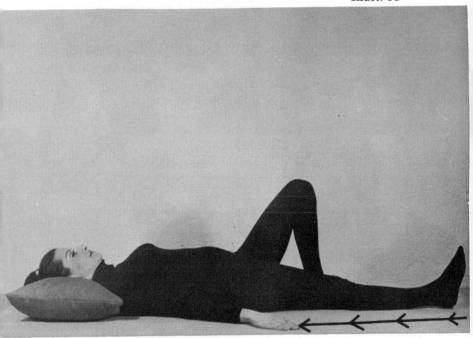

## Exercise 4 (Illust. 61a and 61b)

Relieves fatigue in the cervical and dorsal areas.

**Starting position** Lie on your back, a pillow under your head, draw your knees up over the abdomen and hold them with both hands, inhaling deeply.

a) Raise your head and bend forward so that your forehead is touching your knees. Hold your breath for five seconds

b) Resume starting position, while exhaling.

Four times for beginners, eight for others.

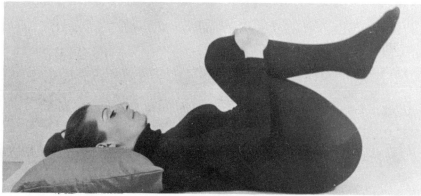

**Illust. 61a**

**Illust. 61b**

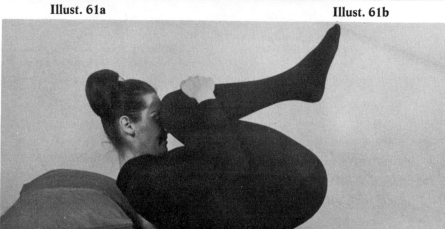

### Exercise 5 (Illust. 62a and 62b)

Strengthens dorsal, abdominal and thigh muscles.

**Starting position**  Lie on your back without a pillow, knees bent, feet together on the floor. Stretch out your arms on each side of your body, palms on the floor.

a) Raise your buttocks as high as possible off the floor so that only your shoulders and feet remain touching the floor. Inhale. Hold this position for five seconds.

b) Return slowly to starting position, exhaling.

Four times for beginners, eight for others.

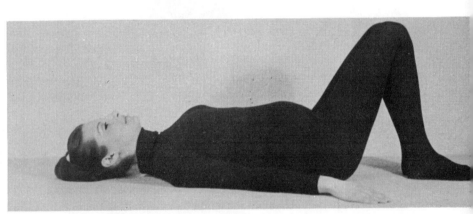

Illust. 62a

Illust. 62b

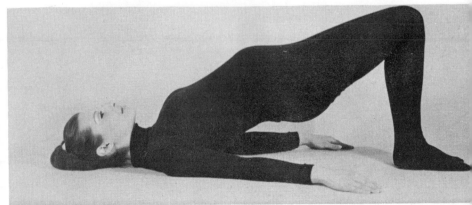

### Exercise 6 (Illust. 63)

Relieves pain in the back and cervical region.

**Starting position**  Sit in a chair or on a stool, with your back straight and your hands at your side.

Make a circular movement with your shoulders, inhaling on one circle, exhaling on the next.

Four times for beginners, eight for others.

**Illust. 63**

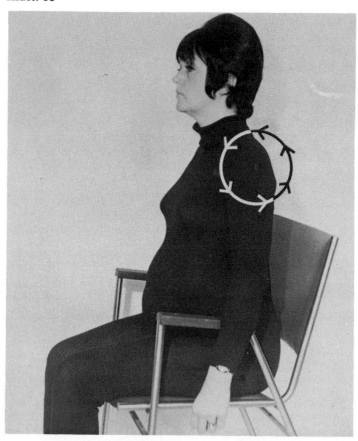

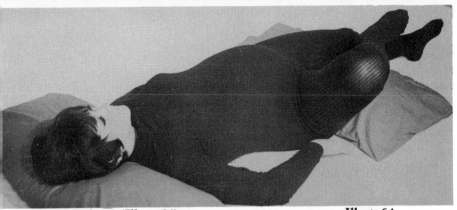

**Exercise 7 (Illust. 64)**

Eliminates strain in the groin area and makes the pelvic joints supple.

**Starting position** Lie on your back, a pillow under your head, another under your thighs, your hands at your side, palms on the floor.

a) Bend your knee slightly to the side, your thigh touching your abdomen, and inhale.

b) Stretch the leg out straight, without pointing the toes, and exhale.

c) Change legs and repeat.

Four times for beginners, eight for others.

**Exercise 8 (Illust. 65a, 65b, 65c)**

Strengthens pelvic and abdominal muscles and relaxes the lumbar-sacral region.

**Starting position** Lie on the floor, a pillow under your head, both arms bent at the elbow, at shoulder height, the lumbar region pressed against the floor.

a) Roll the pelvis to the left, so that your knees are half-way between the floor and the starting position, inhaling.

b) Repeat the exercise, rolling the pelvis to the right, exhaling. Do not allow the knees to touch the floor during this exercise. The resultant twisting motion of the pelvis would be too severe.

Four times for beginners, eight for others.

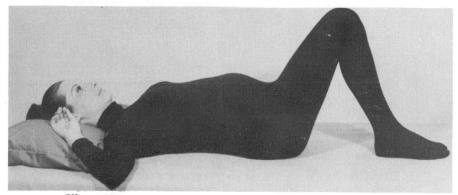

**Illust. 65a**

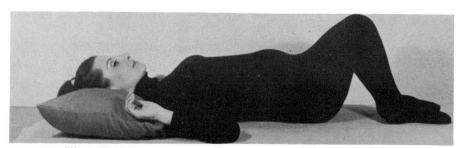

**Illust. 65b**

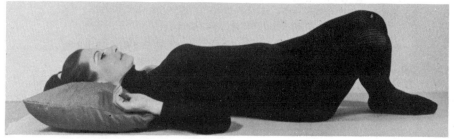

**Illust. 65c**

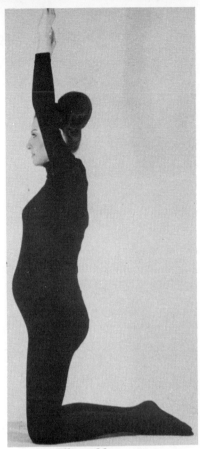

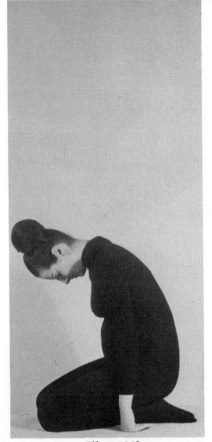

Illust. 66a                    Illust. 66b

### Exercise 9 (Illust. 66a and 66b)

Makes the joints supple and relaxes the spine and alleviates constipation. This is an excellent exercise to stimulate the major vital functions because it brings into play a large number of muscles.

**Starting position**  Sit on your heels, your arms at your sides.

a) Raise your arms and stretch, inhaling.
b) Sit back on your heels, lowering arms and letting your head drop forward, exhaling.

Four times for beginners, eight for others.

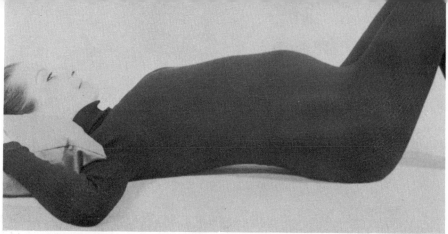

**Illust. 67a**

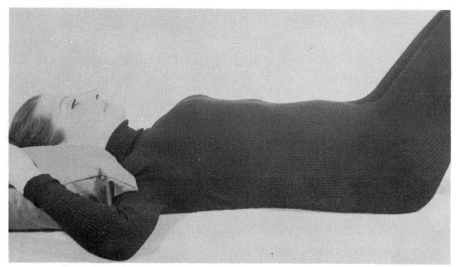

**Exercise 10 (Illust. 67a and 67b)**        **Illust. 67b**

Pelvic rocking.

**Starting position**  Lie on the floor, arms at shoulder level, elbows bent, knees bent, feet flat on the floor.

a) Rock the pelvis while arching the lumbar region. Inhale, pushing out the abdomen.

b) Contract the abdominal muscles, pressing the lumbar area against the floor, while exhaling.

Four times for beginners, eight for others.

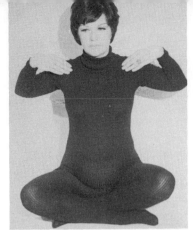

Illust. 68a

Illust. 68c

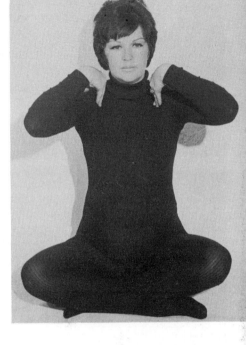

Illust. 68b

### Exercise 11 (Illust. 68a, 68b, 68c)

Because the size of your breasts will increase during pregnancy, it is important to strengthen the pectoral muscles which support them.

**Starting position** Sit in the "tailor" position, your hands on your shoulders.

a) Move your elbows in a circular motion, forwards. Make one circle while inhaling and one circle while exhaling.

b) Repeat, moving the elbows in a circular motion backwards. One circle while ·inhaling, one circle while exhaling.

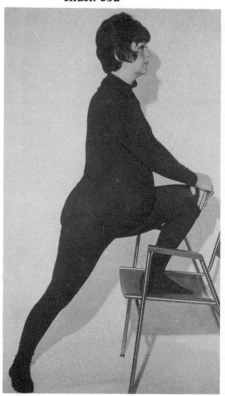 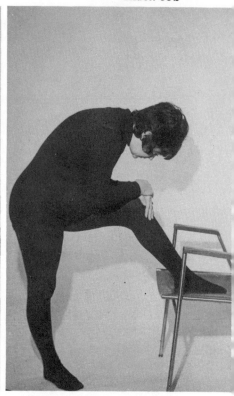

c) Contract your abdominal muscles while inhaling.

Four times for beginners, eight for others.

### Exercise 12  (Illust. 69a and 69b)

Relieves tension in the lumbar region and groin.

**Starting position**  Stand with your left foot on a chair, both hands resting on your knee.

a) Bend the knee and lean forward until your thigh touches your calf while inhaling.

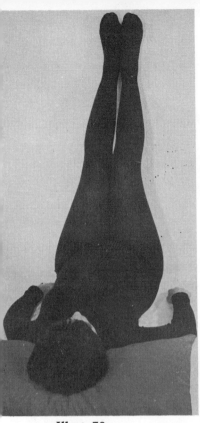

Illust. 70a

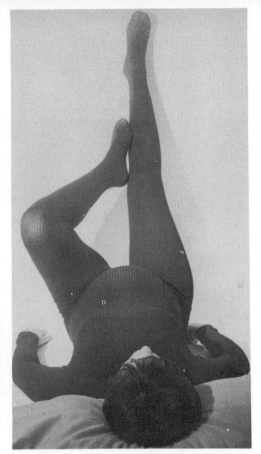

Illust. 70b

b) Return to the starting position, arching your back and allowing your head to fall forward, while exhaling.

Four times for beginners, eight for others.

### Exercise 13 (Illust. 70a, 70b, 70c, 70d)

Leg exercises — especially beneficial to those with varicose veins.

**Starting position** Lie on your back, feet against the wall if you are less than six months pregnant or on a chair if more than six months.

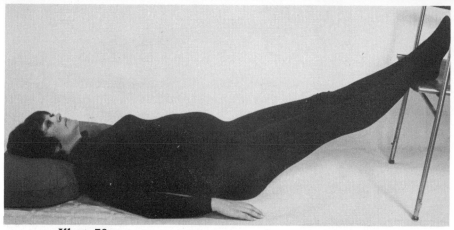

**Illust. 70c**

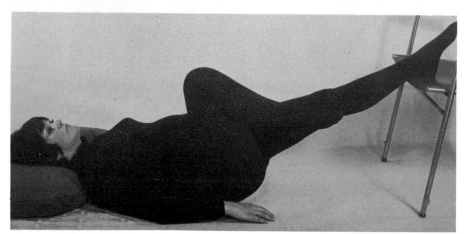

**Illust. 70d**

This position is good for circulation.

Bend one leg, the knee to the outside of the body. Flex the knee joint and place the foot against the wall or chair again while inhaling.

Do this exercise ten times for each leg, changing legs each time. If you close your eyes while performing it, you will find it easy to relax.

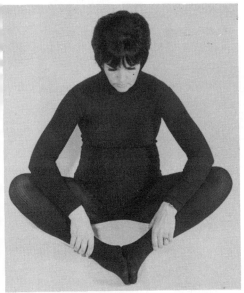

Illust. 71a

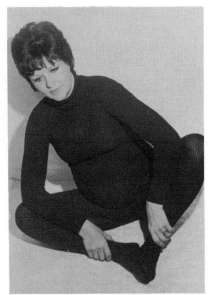

Illust. 71b

### Exercise 14 (Illust. 71a and 71b)

Tones the perinium, facilitates delivery.

**Starting position,** Sit with knees bent, soles of feet together, elbows resting on knees, hands holding the ankles.

a) Press your right elbow against your knee, pushing it down to the floor while inhaling.

b) Repeat on the left side, while exhaling.

Four times for beginners, eight for others.

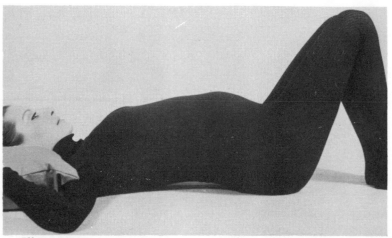

**Illust. 72a**

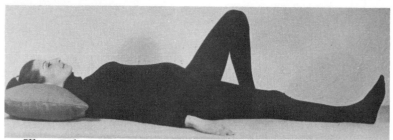

**Illust. 72b**

### Exercise 15 (Illust. 72a and 72b)

Strengthens the abdominal muscles.

**Starting position** Lie on the floor with a pillow under your head, knees bent, feet flat on the floor.

a) Arch the small of the back, pushing out the stomach while inhaling.

b) Stretch your right leg out straight, without pointing the toes. Press the small of your back against the floor and contract the abdominal muscles while exhaling.

Four times for beginners, eight for others.

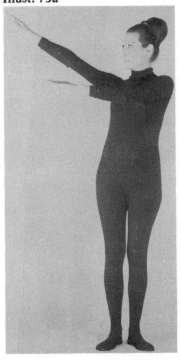
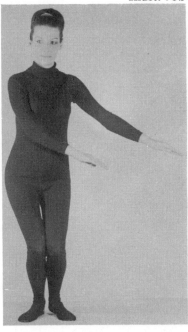

### Exercise 16 (Illust. 73a, 73b)

Relaxes the joints.

**Starting position** Stand with your feet slightly apart, your weight on your right leg.

a) Swing both arms to the right at shoulder height while inhaling.

b) Swing your arms down and then up to the left to shoulder height, bending your knees, transferring your weight to your left foot and exhaling as you do so.

c) Swing your arms back to the right, bending your knees and transferring your weight back to the right foot while inhaling.

Four times for beginners, eight for others.

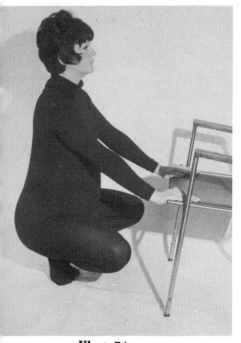

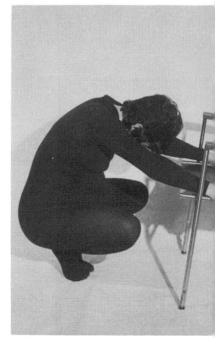

Illust. 74a                        Illust. 74b

### Exercise 17  (Illust. 74a and 74b)

Strengthens the pelvic muscles and prevents constipation.

**Starting position**  Squat down on your haunches, holding on to the seat of a chair.

a) Keeping your back straight, push out your abdomen, while inhaling.

b) Arch your back, letting your head fall forward and contract your abdominal muscles while exhaling.

Four times for beginners, eight for others.

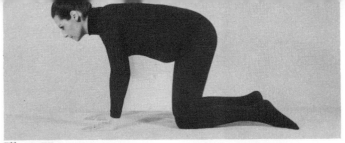

Illust. 75a

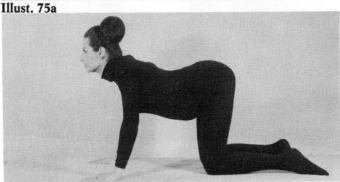

Illust. 75b

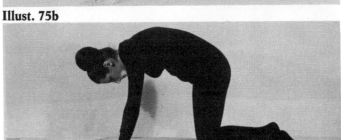

Illust. 75c

### Exercise 18 (Illust. 75a and 75b)

Alleviates backache.

**Starting position** On hands and knees, back perfectly straight, knees slightly apart, abdominal muscles relaxed.

a) Hollow your back by raising your head and buttocks while inhaling.

b) Arch your back by letting your head fall forward and contracting your abdominal muscles while exhaling.

Four times for beginners, eight for others.

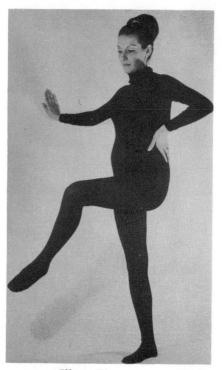

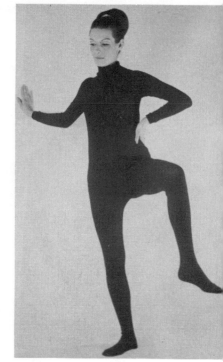

Illust. 76a

Illust. 76b

### Exercise 19 (Illust. 76a and 76b)

Relaxes the muscles of the legs, improves circulation and alleviates pain in the groin, which may occur around the eighth month of pregnancy.

**Starting position**   Stand with your right hand on a wall.

a) With the knee slightly bent, swing your left leg towards the wall while exhaling.

b) In the same position, swing your leg towards the outside while exhaling.

c) Repeat, with right leg.

Four times for beginners, eight for others.

110

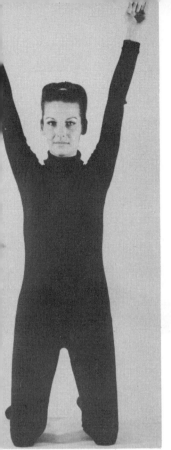

Illust. 77a

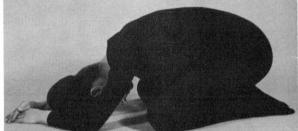

Illust. 77b

**Exercise 20  (Illust. 77a and 77b)**

Strengthens the back.

**Starting position**   Kneeling, knees slightly apart.

a)  Stretch your arms over your head while inhaling.

b)  Lower your arms and head to the ground while exhaling.

Four times for beginners, eight for others.

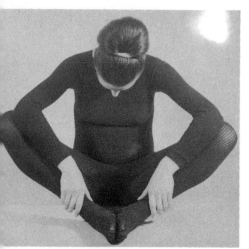

Illust. 78a

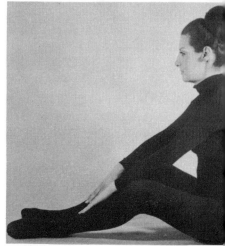

Illust. 78b

### Exercise 21 (Illust. 78a and 78b)

Strengthens the perineum.

**Starting position**  Seated, legs bent, soles of feet touching, hands grasping ankles.

a) Draw your heels as near as possible to your body while inhaling.

b) Stretch your legs out while exhaling.

Four times for beginners, eight for others.

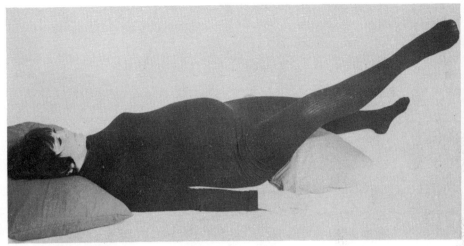

**Illust. 79**

### Exercise 22 (Illust. 79)

Relaxes the groin muscles.

**Starting position**  Lie on your back, a pillow under your head, another under your thighs.

a)  Raise your right leg and swing it to the right while inhaling and towards the left while exhaling.

b)  Change legs and repeat.

Four times for beginners, eight for others.

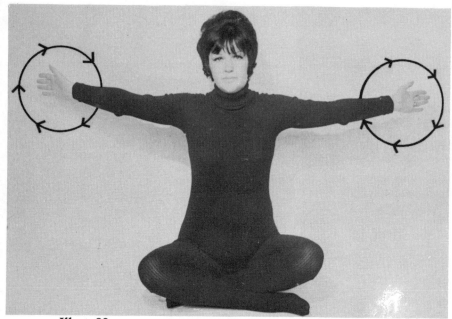

**Illust. 80**

**Exercise 23  (Illust. 80)**

Firms the breasts.

**Starting position**   Sit in the "tailor" position, arms extended to the side at shoulder height.

a) Execute a circling motion with your arms, inhaling while making one circle, exaling while making the next.

Four times for beginners, eight for others.

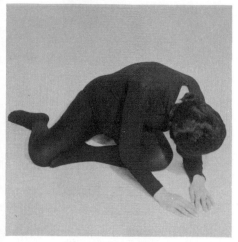

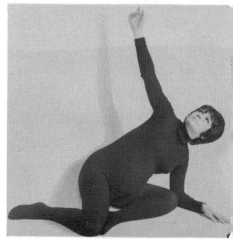

Illust. 81a

Illust. 81b

### Exercise 24 (Illust. 81a and 81b)

Relieves strain in the dorsal-lumbar region of the back and encourages relaxation.

**Starting position**   Sit on the floor, right leg extended behind you and to the right side, knee bent. Left leg bent in front of you, foot against the right thigh.

a) Bend your trunk forward, palms of hands on the floor, head bending towards your left knee.

b) Raise your right arm above your head and, following your hand with your eyes, inhale.

c) Let your head and right arm drop towards the floor, arching your back and exhaling.

Four times for beginners, eight for others.

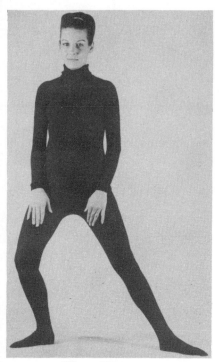

**Illust. 82a**

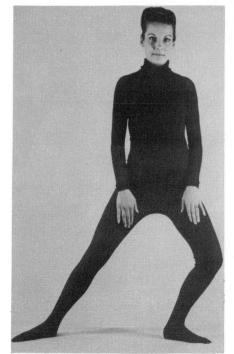

**Illust. 82b**

**Exercise 25 (Illust. 82a and 82b)**

Relaxes the muscles involved in delivery.

**Starting position** Stand with legs two feet apart, toes pointing forwards, hands on thighs.

a) Bend right knee, stretching the muscles of the left leg while inhaling.

b) Bend left knee, stretching the muscles of the right leg while exhaling.

Four times for beginners, eight for others.

116

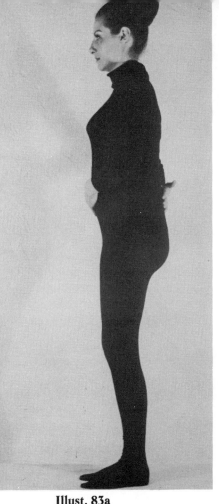
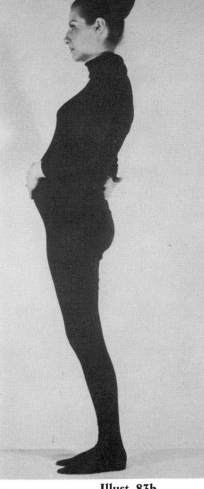

**Illust. 83a**

**Illust. 83b**

**Exercise 26 (Illust. 83 a and 83b)**

Alleviates pain in the lumbar-sacral region.

**Starting position**    Standing, feel slightly apart to maintain balance.

a) Rock the pelvis forward while inhaling. The stomach will protrude and a hollow is formed in the small of the back.

b) Rock pelvis backward while exhaling, contracting the muscles of the abdomen and buttocks.

Four times for beginners, eight for others.

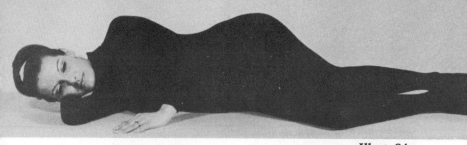

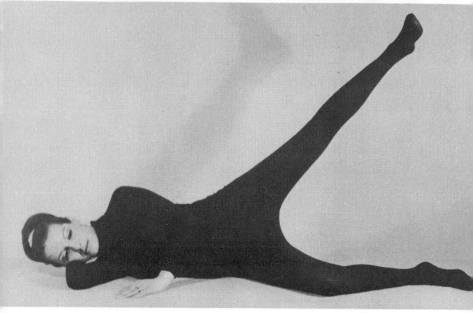

Illust. 84b

### Exercise 27  (Illust. 84a and 84b)

Alleviates constipation.

**Starting position**  Lie on your left side, your head resting on your bent arm, right hand on the floor in front of you to maintain balance.

a)  Raise your left leg while inhaling.

b)  Lower your left leg while exhaling.

c)  Turn on your other side and repeat with right leg.

Four times for beginners, eight for others.

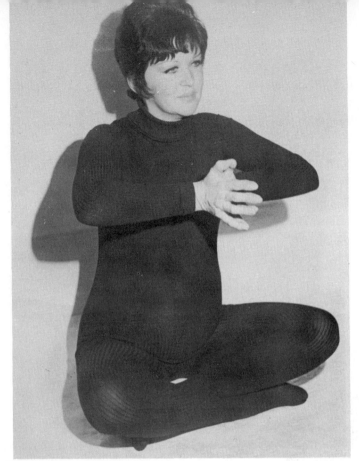

**Illust. 85**

**Exercise 28 (Illust. 85)**

Firms the pectoral muscles.

**Starting position** Sit in the "tailor" position, arms raised, elbows bent, on a level with your breast, palms together, fingers spread.

a)  Press palms together hard while inhaling.

b)  Relax the pressure while exhaling.

Four times for beginners, eight for others.

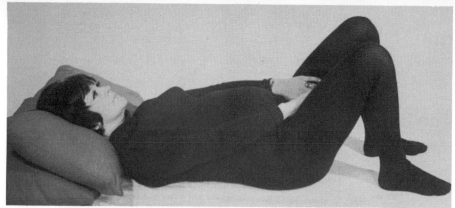

**Illust. 86a**

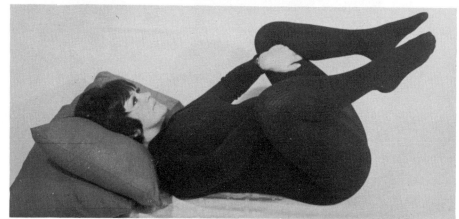

**Illust. 86b**

### Exercise 29 (Illust. 86a and 86b)

Strengthens the abdominal muscles in preparation for delivery.

**Starting position** Lie on the floor, two pillows under your head, knees bent, feet flat on the floor, palms resting on the inside of your thighs.

a) Tighten abdominal muscles while inhaling, pulling your knees towards you.

b) Return to original position while inhaling.

Four times for beginners, eight for others.

## Exercise 30 (Illust. 87a, 87b and 87c)

Strengthens and relaxes the lumbar and abdominal muscles which support the weight of the uterus.

**Starting position**   On hands and knees, back straight, knees apart.

a) Swing the whole trunk forward, leaning on your hands while inhaling.

b) Move back until you are sitting on your heels while exhaling.

From the fourth to the seventh month, repeat this movement ten times before retiring. From the seventh to the ninth month, ten times in mid-morning and ten times in the late afternoon, for a total of twenty times each day.

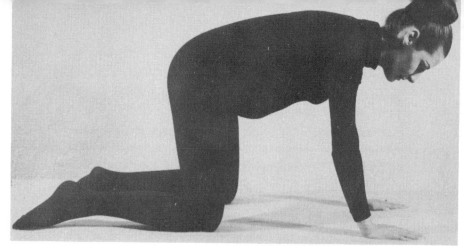

**Illust. 87a**

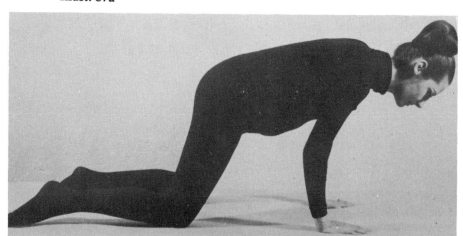

**Illust. 87b**

**Illust. 87c**

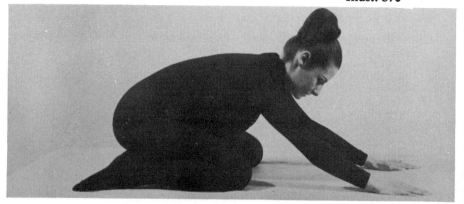

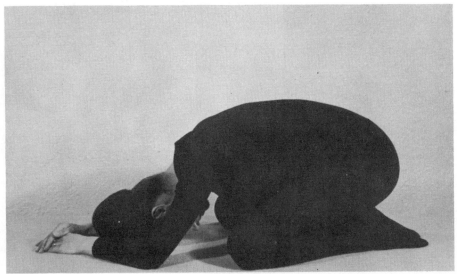

**Illust. 88**

### Exercise 31 (Illust. 88)

Use this "Frog Position" to relax between exercises.

**Starting position** On hands and knees, hands crossed, palms on floor, knees as far apart as possible.

a) Swing the trunk forward until your head is resting on your arms, rest your buttocks on your heels. Hold this position for ten seconds.
If you are unaccustomed to exercise, you may feel a pulling sensation in the hips, groin and thighs.

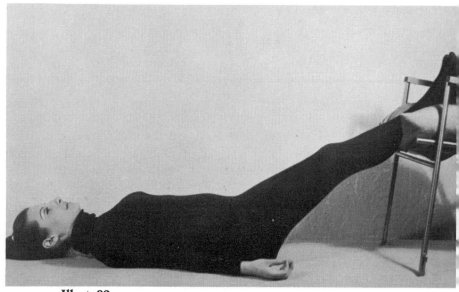

Illust. 89

**Some suggestions for relieving varicose veins and improving circulation.**

a) Place pillows under the foot of your mattress when sleeping.

b) Place three or four books under one end of a folded ironing board.
Stretch out on it, your feet at the elevated end. Relax completely in this position for five minutes.

c) Before retiring, rest your feet on the seat of a chair or against a wall for ten minutes.

# Chapter VI

## Your Anatomy

### The Pelvis and Genital Organs

1. **The bony pelvis** The pelvic girdle, or pelvis, is a bony canal. Its purpose is to protect the internal reproduction organs such as the uterus, the fallopian tubes, the ovaries and the vagina. The pelvis provides a base for the trunk and its top rim is the hip bone. It is formed by three bones, joined by three joints; the two iliac bones, which form the hips, and the sacrum which ends at the coccyx. Two of these joints are called "sacroiliacs" and attach the iliac bones to the sacrum at the hips. The third joint is the "pubic symphysis" which lies under the hairy area of the pubis. It is only during pregnancy that the uterus projects beyond the hip bones. A normal delivery is only possible if your pelvis is of normal size. If during pelvimetry (X-ray of the pelvis) the doctor diagnoses a pelvic malformation, you will probably have to have a Caesarian section. (See Chapter II)

A normally shaped pelvis is called "gynecoid" (in the form of a heart). (Diagram 5)

A pelvis could be "platypelloid" (flat), or "anthropoid" (long and narrow). (Diagram 6)

During pregnancy, many changes occur. The ligaments and joints permit the pelvic cavity to enlarge in order to facilitate the passage of the baby.

### The Perineum

2. **The Soft Pelvis** The soft pelvis is formed by muscles which are called the "perineum" or pelvic floor. The perineum covers three orifices. (Diagram 7)

125

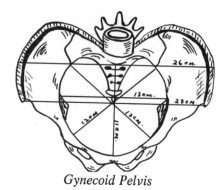

*Gynecoid Pelvis*

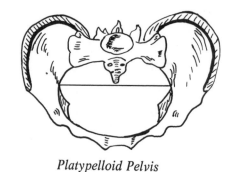

*Platypelloid Pelvis*

**Diagram 5**

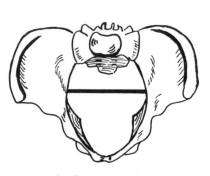

*Anthropoid Pelvis*

**Diagram 6**

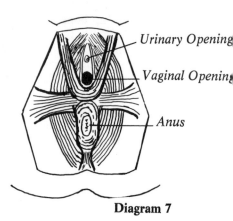

Urinary Opening

Vaginal Opening

Anus

**Diagram 7**

- the urinary opening, which leads to the bladder.
- the vagina, which leads to the neck of the uterus.
- the anus, which leads to the rectum.

**The Reproductive Organs**

**The Uterus,** more commonly known as the "womb". This is a firm, pear-shaped muscular organ which rests in an upside-down position in the pelvis. The body or main part

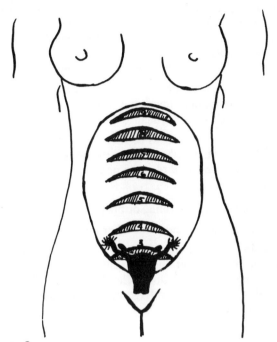

**Diagram 8**

of the uterus is approximately two inches long and the neck
or cervix, is approximately one to one and a half inches
long. The cervix extends into the vagina. The bottom of
the uterus (or the large part of the pear) rises into the abdominal area as the pregnancy progresses. (Diagram 8)

During the pregnancy, the interwoven elastic fibres of the
uterus allow it to dilate. During the last stage of pregnancy,
these muscular fibres contract and stretch in a regular
manner to permit the cervix to dilate. This is called **labour.**

Except during pregnancy, the vaginal opening is the size of a straw and allows sperm to enter and the menstrual flow to drain. In the course of a birth, this opening enlarges as a result of regular contractions to approximately four inches in diameter to provide a passage for the baby.

At the top, on each side, the uterus is extend by two passages called **fallopian tubes**, the ends of which cover the **ovaries** like a cap with a fringe.

During pregnancy the uterus contains the fetus, the placenta, the umbilical cord, membranes and the amniotic fluid. Therefore, labour is comprised of three phases:

1. Dilation of the cervix.

2. The expulsion of the fetus, or birth.

3. Delivery of the placenta and other parts.

**The Vagina** is like an elastic sheath which stretches to allow passage of the baby at the moment of delivery, much the same as it permits copulation. The dimensions of the vagina are variable and it can undergo great distension, especially during delivery.


### Intra-Uterine Life

In the uterus, the fetus receives the nourishment and oxygen which it needs to develop by means of the placenta and umbilical cord. (Diagram 9) These are temporary organs and become useless after birth.

**The Placenta** is vital to the life of the fetus and resembles a spongy mass. It adheres to one side of the uterine wall — this is termed the maternal surface of the placenta. The fetal surface is the side facing the fetus and is quite different in appearance. The placenta provides oxygen and all the other substances which are indispensable to the development of the fetus. These substances are transferred to the baby by way of the umbilical cord. The placenta serves the fetus as lungs, stomach, intestines and kidneys throughout its uterine life.

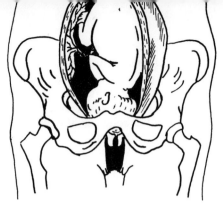

*The position of the fetus at term*

**Diagram 9**

The ratio of the weight of the placenta to the weight of the fetus is about 1 to 6. In other words, if the fetus weighs six pounds, the placenta weighs an average of one pound.

**The Umbilical Cord**   The placenta is attached to the fetus by the umbilical cord. It contains three blood vessels — a large central vessel (the umbilical vein) and two smaller vessels (the umbilical arteries). These three blood vessels are coiled around each other in a spiral and surrounded by a gelatinous membrane. Contrary to the usual pattern, the vein carries nutritious maternal blood to the fetus and the fetal blood, containing wastes and carbon dioxide is discharged into the maternal circulation by the two arteries. The role of the cord is essentially that of a conductor. After the birth of the baby, as soon as he has begun to breathe and has emitted his first cry, the cord is cut. It is then that the baby becomes independent. The cord measures from twenty to forty inches and is about the size of the little finger.

**The Membranes**   Nourished by the placenta and fed by the umbilical cord, the fetus is protected by two cloaks which are called "membranes". The outer cloak is the *chorion,* the inner is the *amnion.* The membranes resemble a plastic bag. The amnion secretes a clear liquid which surrounds the fetus. This is the amniotic fluid or the "water". Its role is to protect and isolate the fetus from the outside. The membranes, having neither blood or nerve supply, rupture painlessly. They can rupture spontaneously before the beginning of contractions, during labour, or the doctor can rupture them in order to start contractions.

**The Amniotic Fluid**  The fetus is bathed in this fluid which keeps it at a constant temperature. It also holds the walls of the uterus apart so that the baby will not be bothered by the uterine muscle. As a fluid, it cannot be compressed and prevents shock. If the mother falls, the fetus is well protected. However, if the shock is violent, the risk is more serious. A great part of the amniotic fluid is provided by the urine of the fetus. This urine is sterile since the fetus returns all wastes by way of the placenta. The fluid is renewed several times a day. The fetus swallows a certain amount and he urinates it, but it is clean and inoffensive. The normal quantity is about one pint. If the fluid is excessive (approvimately two pints) the condition is called "hydramnios".

## The Development of the Fetus in the Uterus

### The First Month

The union of the sperm and ovum forms a mass of small cells which at the end of four days penetrates into the upper part of the uterus. (Diagram 10) This cluster of cells attaches itself to the wall of the uterus, causing the rupture of some blood vessels. This is called the implantation of the egg.

**Diagram 10**

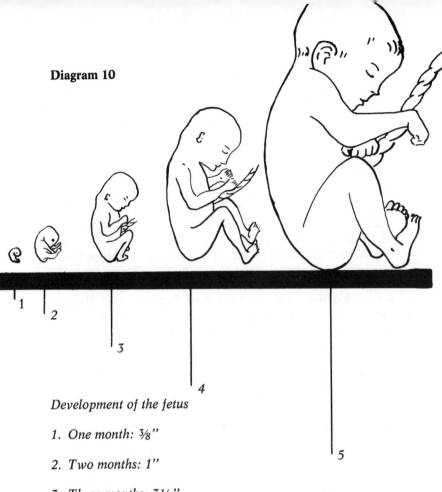

*Development of the fetus*

1. *One month: ⅜"*

2. *Two months: 1"*

3. *Three months: 3½"*

4. *Four months: 6¼"*

5. *Six months: 11⅞"*

At the end of the second week the cluster of cells has formed an embryo. This causes menstruation to cease. The production of a certain hormone suppresses ovulation and this continues until the end of pregnancy. At the end of twenty-seven days, the placenta, attached to one side of the uterine wall, begins to carry out its function. The embryo at this period is perfectly formed from head to toe. The heart begins to beat around the twenty-second day, but is too faint to be heard with a stethoscope. At thirty days the embryo is the size of a pea, or ten thousand times larger than the fertile ovum.

## The Second Month

By the middle of the second month, the embryo is about one inch long, but is so light it can hardly be weighed. The head has increased in size and is about as large as the rest of the body. The embryo begins to turn its head, to close its mouth and to swallow the amniotic fluid. The eyes, nose, ears, lips, tongue and roots of the milk teeth develop. Its body is padded with incipient muscle and is covered with a very thin skin. The arms are short, but the hands already have a thumb and fingers. The central nervous system is growing rapidly. When the embryo has reached this stage without accident or disease, it has a good start in life and is ready to enter into another stage in its development. It is inadvisable for the pregnant woman to receive X-rays at this time since they could hinder the development of the fetus.

## The Third Month

Toward the middle of the third month, the future mother will notice that her clothes are beginning to feel tight. The uterus has begun to increase in order to accommodate a fetus which is now three to four inches in length. This is the point at which the embryo becomes a fetus.

Teeth are forming under the gums and the eyes have lids which now fuse and do not re-open until the sixth month. The ears shape and the feet begin to develop. The fetus begins to move its legs and feet, to clench its fist, to squint, to frown, to open its mouth and purse its lips. At the beginning of the third month, the genital organs take shape. Although the sex of the child has been determined at the moment of conception, until this time the embryo has had both male and female organs.

## The Fourth Month

Sometime during this month you will probably feel the baby's first movements, as the tiny body rocks back and forth. This is a month of refinements, some of them of an aesthetic nature. The features of the face are completed. The eyes, which were far from the nose, draw closer together, the eyelids form and the skin becomes covered with fine hair.

The heart beats very quickly, twice as fast as that of an adult. The digestive tract begins to function (gall bladder and stomach) and in the intestines a green substance called "meconium" accumulates. The kidneys also function. Urine is spilled into the amniotic fluid. Hair begins to grow. The size of the fetus increases from four to seven inches in length and its weight from one ounce to eight ounces. If it continued to grow at the same rate, it would weigh nearly 250 pounds at birth!

The increased rate of growth is due to the increase in the size of the placenta. The nutrient elements, water and oxygen, reach the placenta in the blood and are transported to the fetus by the umbilical cord, while wastes are removed. The blood of the mother and fetus do not mix. The maternal blood flow penetrates the placenta and the nutritive elements it contains proceed into the blood vessels of the cord to nourish the fetus. The wastes pass from the fetus to the placenta and from there into the mother's blood. In this way, the cord transports approximately thirty pints of liquid in both directions each day.

## The Fifth Month

By this time the fetus has begun to move a great deal, especially when you are resting. The small, fluttery movement of the fourth month soon become much stronger. Floating in the amniotic fluid, he jumps, kicks, an even turns sommersaults. Periods of rest alternate with periods of activity. When he sleeps, he assumes his favorite position, all curled up. He can be disturbed by external noises. Loud music, the vibration of the washing machine, his mother bumping into something, can awaken him and lead to a period of activity. He begins to suck his thumb and will do so throughout the period of inter-uterine life.

He measures ten to twelve inches and weighs about one pound. His length will have doubled by the time of birth. His weight gradually increases, and during the last three months reaches a total of six to nine pounds.

## The Sixth Month

The development of the muscles is signified by increased movement. The fetus makes about 200 movements a day. The skin is markedly wrinkled, but there is a beginning deposit of fat beneath it. The doctor can hear the heartbeat with his stethoscope and if there are twins, he may hear two. The mother will begin to recognize the different parts of the baby's body. By feeling the movements of her abdomen, she can distinguish the hands from the feet and the head from the bottom. Sometimes she will notice regular movements at intervals of fifteen to thirty seconds. These are hiccups, caused by the fetus swallowing the amniotic fluid. The fetus now weighs about one-and-a-half pounds and measures from eleven to fourteen inches. Because he is floating in the amniotic fluid, the mother does not experience the sensation of carrying this much weight. Also because of this buoyancy, the fetus is able to turn in a way that will be impossible for him after birth until he is several months old. His skin is protected against injury by a thick layer of whitish cream, not unlike that used by long distance swimmers. This fatty coating is called "vernix caseosa" or sebum.

## The Seventh Month

By this time his hair is quite long and the fine hair which covered his body is already starting to disappear. He looks like a little old man with reddish, wrinkled skin, devoid of fat. He weighs about three pounds and is from fourteen to sixteen inches long. An infant this size is very immature, but his organs are sufficiently developed to make his chances for survival reasonably good if he were delivered at this point.

## The Eight Month

During the last two months a layer of fat is produced which acts as a padding and which will keep his body warm after birth. If the mother overeats, the baby will also be fat. He is so large that the uterus is crowded and he is not able to move around with as much freedom. He will probably rest with his head downwards. Most babies adopt this position, probably because the head weighs more than the rest of the body and also because the shape of the head adapts well to the rounded form of the base of the uterus. The main organs are now functioning perfectly. The wrinkles disappear and the reddish tint of the skin fades to pink. If delivered at this stage, he would have a very good chance of surviving without difficulty. He weighs from four to five pounds and is about eighteen inches long.

## The Ninth Month

During this period the fetus acquires essential immunity against certain illnesses. His lungs are completely developed and the co-ordination of his movements improves. The uterus is now 500 times larger than it was before the pregnancy began.

At some point in the ninth month, a hormone reaction in the mother causes profound changes in the uterine muscle. This is called "labor". In the first stages of this phenomenon, the muscles of the uterus exert a force of fifty pounds per square inch. This force succeeds in expelling the fetus from the cell which he has occupied throughout the pregnancy. He weighs from seven to nine pounds and is from nineteen to twenty-one inches long. Within several hours of his birth, important modifications take place in his system which enable him to adapt to the new surroundings in which he suddenly finds himself.

# Obstetrical Anaesthesia

The unceasing efforts exerted in medicine and related sciences to relieve and even eliminate pain in the human body have met with great success. One branch of medicine in which progress has been constant in anaesthesia. Applied originally to that other discipline, surgery, from which it is inseparable today, it has branched out into other fields. Obstetrics, or the science of pregnancy and delivery, no longer hesitates to make use of anaesthesia.

Anaesthesia is a science which is so diverse that it is impossible to number its applications and its advantages. But there are also some risks and disadvantages. There are many differences between surgical and obstetrical anaesthesia. We will deal here only with the main difference. First of all, obstetrical anaesthesia will affect two subjects, the mother and the child, and each will react in quite a different manner to a given dose. The baby is not able to withstand the same amount of anaesthetic as the mother without risk of noxious effect, such as depression of the respiratory centre which would result in the baby taking longer to breathe spontaneously at birth. If this occurs, resuscitation becomes of vital importance.

One must remember that for a normal childbirth anaesthesia is not essential. If a fatal complication should result from it, the responsibility for a death that could have been avoided would be heavy indeed.

Also, anesthesia must not be allowed to interfere with uterine contractions. It might cause labor to be unduly prolonged, or, after birth, lead to severe hemorrhage due to weakness in the muscle or absence of uterine contractions. In surgical anaesthesia there is ample time to insure proper safeguards; in obstetrical anaesthesia sometimes it is impossible. Labor can start at any time and it might happen that anaesthetic would be administered soon after a meal with the resultant risk of vomiting or aspiration of food into the windpipe.

In spite of whatever hazards may be attached to obstetrical anaesthesia, remember that your doctor will not administer it unless he thinks it is safe — and with modern technique and equipement, there is little risk.

### Regional and Local Anaesthesia

In regional anaesthesia the nerves that carry sensations from the uterus and the pelvic region to the spinal cord are blocked. This may be done by local injection, paracervical nerve block, pudendal block or an epidural block. Some of the agents used for regional anaesthesia are Novocaine, Metycaine, Carbocaine and Xylocaine. If you are likely to have a reaction to one of these products your doctor will inject a small amount of the one he intends to use under the skin on the inside of the forearm before injection, in order to test for sensitivity and allergy .

**Local Injection**   This technique consists simply of injecting a limited zone, such as a small portion of the pirineum where the episiotomy (an incision to enlarge the vaginal orifice) will be made. There are scarcely any risks and the zone of anaesthesia usually remains insensitive for a long enough period of time.

**Paracervical Injection**   In this case the anaesthetic is injected into several points around the neck of the uterus. At the moment of uterine contraction, the force produced by the head of the baby applied on the neck of the uterus in order to dilate it causes pain, especially when dilation reaches the point of three inches. At this point, the anaesthetic is injected. In this case only the neck of the uterus is anaesthetized and if an episiotomy is necessary, a supplementary injection in the area of the perineum will be necessary.

**Pudendal Block**  The injection of a local anaesthetic in the immediate vicinity of the pudendal nerve root blocks the response of the nerve below that site, giving the same effect as if the entire region ennervated by that root were anaesthetized.

The pudendal nerve, which distributes branches to the perineum, the vulva and the vagina, is easily located on the ischial bone of the pelvis during a vaginal examination. It is at this spot that the anaesthetic is injected.

**Epidural Anaesthesia**  The spinal cord distributes different nerves or nerve roots to the whole body. If anaesthetic is injected at a specific point in the spinal column, usually the lumbar region, the same reaction occurs as was discussed above in the pudendal block. However, in this case the anaesthetic works at more nerve root levels; that is, all those nerves which emerge from the spinal cord below the level of the injection are affected. This means that the entire lower part of the body becomes insensitive.

This anaesthesia is administered by an anaesthetist and it presents no major dangers when the technique is well controlled.

There are also a number of other forms of anaesthesia, including caudal and spinal anaesthetics.

To summarize, obstetrical anaesthetic procedures have improved over the years and while general anaesthesia may carry more risks, the development of new local and regional anaesthetic techniques have greatly reduced the hazards to the baby in obstetrical anaesthesia.

Remember that a sedative or other drug taken even very shortly before birth enters the circulatory system of the fetus. Their effect is to reduce the amount of oxygen carried to the baby and act on the respiratory centre of his brain by weakening his desire to breathe. A child born without the use of anaesthetics will be much more active at birth. In almost every case he will breathe spontaneously without the help of the doctor. In cases where anaesthetics are used, the infants are very much more likely to experience respiratory difficulties.

## To Your Husband

The traditional view of division of duties within the family was that the woman underwent pregnancy after pregnancy while dealing at the same time with the education of the children and the internal organization of the home. The husband and father provided the necessary resources needed to maintain the family.

The outlook today is quite different. More and more women work outside the home or are busy with outside interests which provide mental stimulation and satisfaction. Husbands are becoming more involved in the home and in the care and education of their children.

### During Pregnancy

A father who takes no interest in his son until he is old enough to be a companion is being unfair. The nine-month waiting period is a difficult one for the mother and she has the right to expect help and support from her husband. Having read Chapter I, you will understand the enormous changes that occur in your wife's body during pregnancy. Her appetite increases and she will need your encouragement to stick to her diet. She requires a great deal of sleep, at least ten hours a night and you can help by making sure she gets to bed at a reasonable hour every night. While the fun and excitement of an occasional party is good for her and the odd late night will not do any harm, do not make a habit of staying out late every weekend.

You must realize that her prenatal exercises are very important in preparing her for the birth and never make fun of her or tease her about them no matter how strange they seem to you. On the contrary, you should encourage her to do them every day.

There are several things you can do to help your wife which will make her happy and more content.

• Accompany her to the doctor's on her first and last visits. She will appreciate your moral support.

• If she seems particularly nervous or irritable, take her out for the evening to the theatre or to her favorite restaurant.

• Remember that expressions of your love are more important to her now than they every were before.

• Do not remind her constantly of the sex you prefer the child to be. Remember there is a 50% chance that you will get what you want. Also remember that you are responsible for determining the sex of the child!

• Avoid expressing doubts about her ability as a mother — she may be having doubts of her own and she needs reassurance from you.

• Be sympathetic about her fears and worries concerning birth. Encourage her to find the answers to her questions, either from her doctor or from a book like this one. Talk about the things that are worrying her and you will be surprised at how much better she will feel.

A pregnancy is a marvellous work of nature, not something to suffer through passively. A husband and wife who learn together all they can about it will find it an enriching experience.

For the past several years, I have encouraged husbands to share as many aspects of the pregnancy as possible. You can accompany your wife to lectures given at most prenatal clinics, where slides and films are shown which will familiarize you with the process of birth. (Illust. 90) If your wife has decided to have natural childbirth, you will want to accompany her to her classes to learn what to expect.

Some hospitals allow husbands to sit with their wives during the early stages of labor, or even to be present in the delivery rooms. If this is the case, then you will want to be fully prepared for the important role you will be playing in the delivery. The hospitals have classes which explain the mechanics of delivery and the various phases of labor. Here, too, you will be taught to apply certain pressures to your wife's abdomen to help her during labor. (Illust. 91) You and your wife may also be able to visit a delivery room in order to familiarize yourselves with the equipment.

### Labor

If the hospital does allow you to stay with your wife during labor, you can be an enormous help to her by remaining calm and offering encouragement as well as moral and physical support. Although she may not say so at the time, your wife will be very grateful for your help, and she will thank you afterward.

If you have learned the different breathing techniques she must use during labor, you can help by breathing with her. In any case, hold her hand and sponge her forehead with a cool cloth. She may want cool water to rinse her mouth and you can help her with this.

Do not leave the room without warning her and do not chat with the nurse when you think your wife is asleep. Her eyes may be closed, but she certainly is not asleep! Do not talk to her during a contraction, she needs all her concentration to carry out the job at hand.

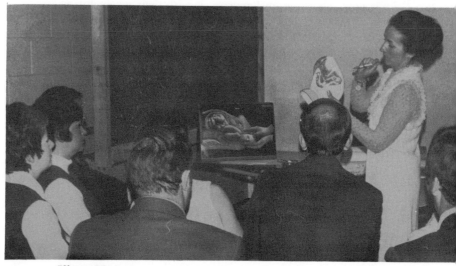

**Illust. 90**

**Illust. 91**

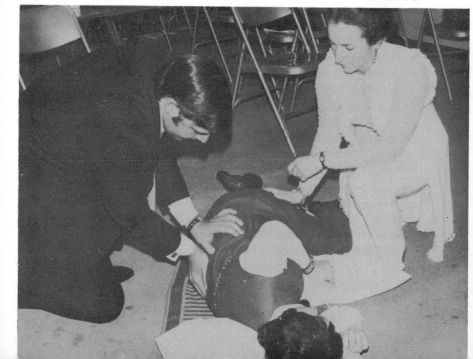

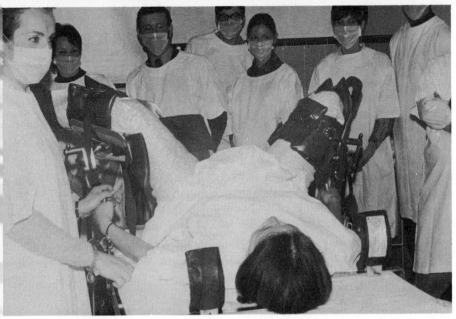

**Illust. 92**

### The Delivery

If the hospital will allow you to be present for the actual delivery, and if your wife wants you to be there, it will be an exciting experience, one which will draw you closer to your wife. However, do not attempt this if you are in any way inclined to be squeamish or if you think the experience will be unsettling. The last thing needed in a delivery room is a fainting father!

You will have little to do but remain quiet and watch. You will be seated where your wife can see you and your presence will be a great comfort to her.

## The Return Home

Your wife will remain in hospital from three to ten days following the birth of child. This time is very pleasant for her in that she may rest, is free of household responsibilty and, best of all, is the centre of your attention.

Except for those mothers who breast feed their babies, the return home may be rather difficult. For the first time, the mother is expected to handle and care for the child she has only held briefly while in the hospital. The first few days may be difficult for all of you, but be patient, a routine will soon be established and life will become reasonably normal.

If you can possibly manage to obtain some help for your wife, this is the time to do so. If not, you will have to help with the housework and take some of the responsibility of night feedings and changings.

Finally. you must understand that it may be several weeks before you and your wife can resume normal sexual relations. This activity can be very painful for your wife, especially if there was any incision made at the time of delivery. It is necessary to wait until she is completely well. Try to remember that this may be almost as difficult for her as it is for you.

Most women are able to return to normal activities from four to six weeks after the delivery. Younger women will recover their strength more quickly. In the meantime, your role as a new father is to be as understanding and helpful as you can.

Pregnancy and birth bring various responsibilities to both partners in the marriage — and many couples have profited from the event to strengthen their union. Certainly, if you are both well prepared and well informed, you will be less likely to have the problems and misunderstandings which are so common during this time.

## Breathing During Labor

There are several breathing techniques taught in connection with natural childbirth. After having given birth to three children by natural childbirth, I no longer believe that it is necessary to know several different breathing methods. When the time comes to use them, one never knows which one to use! I think these techniques for use during labor and delivery are sufficient:

1. Slow, deep breathing during the first contractions until dilation is about five centimeters.

2. Abdominal breathing, gradually becoming faster as the contractions become longer until dilation is about eight centimeters.

3. Superficial breathing or panting until dilation is complete (eleven centimeters).

4. Holding your breath as you push to aid the exit of the fetus.

## False Labor

During the last few weeks of pregnancy, the uterus will harden and remain contracted for several minutes. This will happen at irregular intervals and you may think that labor is beginning.

However, this is not the case. The neck of the uterus is being prepared for the birth by these involuntary contractions. Remember to breathe deeply when you feel the contractions. It has been said that if you experience a great many false contractions, you will have an easy labor.

The fetus benefits from these false contractions also, in that the contractions and relaxation of the muscle aids the development of the lungs. Your baby will therefore breathe more easily when he is delivered.

# The Beginning of Labor

## Characteristic Signs

1. Loss of the mucous plug. This is a gelatinous mass which has been secreted by the cervical glands and which has accumulated in the cervical canal during pregnancy. It has served to close the opening leading to the uterine cavity, as a protective barrier against exterior infection.

2. Some loss of blood.

3. Rupture of the membranes. The membranes containing the amniotic fluid that surrounds the baby (the bag of waters) may break at any time before or during labor. If before, then labor usually begins within twenty-four hours. If labor does not begin, then it is induced by the doctor.

4. Contractions will come at regular intervals and will be quite different from false labor contractions.

The onset of true labor is marked by a dull, low backache and a feeling of tightness in the abdomen. This is soon followed by noticeable uterine contractions which are characterized by an intermittent dragging sensation first in the back then in the lower part of the abdomen and possibly in the thighs. Early labor may be similar to menstrual cramps.

Once labor begins, contractions occur at regular intervals. At first, the contractions are mild and cause little discomfort. They may occur at ten to twenty minute intervals and last from fifteen to thirty seconds. As labor progresses, the contractions gradually increase in intensity and in frequency until they recur every three to four minutes and last from fifty to seventy-five seconds, or even longer.

# Phases of Labor

### 1. Softening of the Cervix or Cervical Effacement

This is the process by which the cervical canal is progressively changed from a structure that is from one to two centimetres long to one so short that it no longer exists.

**Diagram 11**

## SOFTENING OF THE CERVIX

*The cervix has not begun to soften*

*The cervix has begun to soften*

*The softening of the cervix is complete*

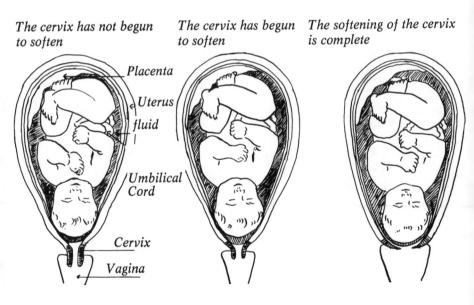

Placenta

Uterus

fluid

Umbilical Cord

Cervix

Vagina

## 2. Dilation

This phase is complete when the dilation of the cervix has progressed from a very small opening to an opening large enough to permit passage of the baby's head.

Be sure to note the time when the contractions began and any other signs which indicate the beginning of labor. When you call the doctor, he will want to know:

1. Whether you have lost any blood
2. Whether the membrane has broken
3. How long you have been having regular contractions
4. The length of time between contractions
5. How long the contractions last

If you can give him accurate answers to these questions, he will be able to judge how far your labor has progressed and when you should go to the hospital.

**Diagram 12**

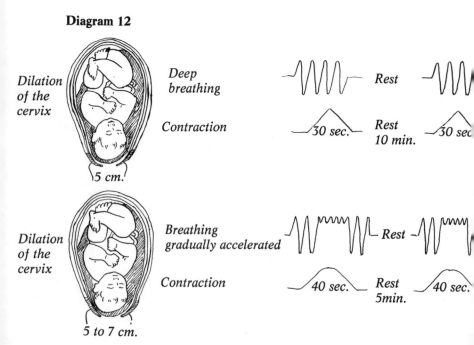

The second phase of labor, dilation, is further divided into three stages.

**First Stage** Dilation from ½ centimeter up to five centimeters. (Diagram 12) This stage can last from five to eight hours for a woman having her first child. It is much faster with a woman who has had one or more children. The contractions are not very close together, nor are they particularly intense. You may want to move around between contractions. During the contraction, you will breathe deeply, distending your abdomen.

**Second Stage** Dilation from five to seven centimeters. (Diagram 12)

For a first child, this stage will last from two to three hours. Contractions will be stronger and last longer — from forty-five to sixty seconds. The intervals will be from four to five minutes long.

You will breathe slowly and deeply, gradually accelerating at the height of the contraction.

**Diagram 13**

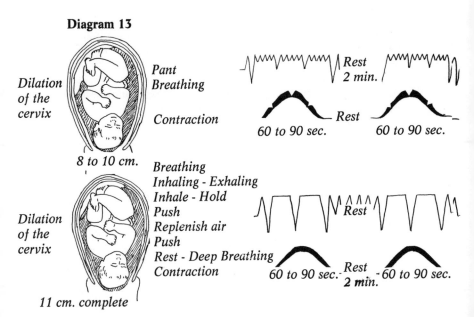

Dilation of the cervix

Pant Breathing

Contraction

Rest 2 min.

60 to 90 sec.    Rest    60 to 90 sec.

8 to 10 cm.

Dilation of the cervix

Breathing
Inhaling - Exhaling
Inhale - Hold
Push
Replenish air
Push
Rest - Deep Breathing
Contraction

Rest

60 to 90 sec.    Rest 2 min.    60 to 90 sec.

11 cm. complete

**Third Stage**   Dilation from seven to eleven centimeters. (Diagram 13)

This stage lasts from thirty to sixty minutes and completes the dilation for passage of the child. You will be fairly uncomfortable during this time, and may notice several disagreeable symptoms. You may experience nausea, or even vomiting. This possibility is why you are advised not to take any solid food after labor begins. In the case of an anaesthetic being used during the later stages of labor, food could be aspirated into the bronchial tubes.

You may feel restless and even shiver. This is a nervous reaction and can be alleviated by relaxing as much as possible and breathing in short, quick pants.

Some women find that their teeth chatter and their legs shake. These, too, are nervous reactions and one best relieved by relaxing and concentrating on your breathing exercises.

You may feel an irresistable desire to push at this stage — but you must not do so. The fetus exerts a strong pressure on the cervix and you will feel that you should push. However, you should not do so until the doctor tells you to (until dilation is complete).

Premature pushing may well delay the delivery because if the dilation is not sufficient, you may tear the opening. In some cases, the mother does not feel the desire to push. This may be because the uterine contractions were not long enough, or the fetus was wrongly presented. In any case, this period before complete dilation may pass quickly for a mother who does not feel the desire to push.

**Panting or Superficial Breathing**

This breathing technique is very useful during the latter stages of labor as the diaphragm moves very little and does not interfere with the uterine contractions. The rapid breathing helps increase the supply of oxygen to the uterine muscles when it is most needed.

This breathing is done through the mouth, inhaling only a little air at a time and exhaling immediately. Deep breaths are interspersed at short intervals. Try not to open your mouth too far since the membranes inside the mouth will dry quickly and become uncomfortable. Tuck your tongue behind your lower teeth and keep your lips just slightly parted. This will stimulate the saliva glands and ensure sufficient moisture. Some hospitals provide cracked ice which is refreshing; others provide water or other liquids.

Panting uses only the top parts of the lungs and is clearly audible. The abdomen may move, but this is normal. You may feel dizzy or a choking sensation after a few moments of superficial breathing. This is due to the increase of oxygen and is quite normal. The fetus may increase its movements for the same reason. You should not begin this rapid breathing too soon to avoid becoming tired.

**Steps to Follow**   At the beginning of the contraction

- take a deep breath
- exhale deeply
- take ten short, rapid breaths.

This will take about five seconds.  Then,

- take a deep breath
- take ten shallow, rapid breaths.

Continue in this manner until the contraction begins to ease. Then,

- exhale deeply.

- inhale deeply

When you are used to it, lengthen the rhythm of your breathing to adapt it to the intensity of the contraction. In short, the stronger the contraction, the quicker the breathing.

### Exercise - 90 seconds

- inhale deeply

- exhale deeply

- breathe through your mouth, accelerating the rhythm like a train as it picks up speed

- continue for ten to fifteen seconds, then exhale deeply

- repeat from the beginning

Remember that you should always take a deep breath at the end of a contraction.

Practise this method of breathing in different positions — sitting down, lying on your back, and on your side. You should practise until you can breathe in this manner for ninety seconds — the average length of a contraction in the third stage of dilation.

### Massage of the Abdomen

During contractions, the skin of the abdomen will become very tender and sensitive. Light massage with the fingertips will ease the tension and provide a soothing sensation. If you adopt a regular rhythm for this massage and breathe according to the intensity of the contraction, you will feel very much better.

To practise this massage at home, lie flat on your back, a pillow under your head, knees bent and lightly massage the skin of your stomach with a rotating movement. (Illust. 93) Begin with the fingers of both hands touching at the pubic area, move outward toward your hips and then inward toward your navel. Then reverse the motion. Remember to use only very light pressure, since too much pressure will stimulate the uterine muscles.

**Massage Exercises Adapted to Different Breathing Methods**

**"Long, deep" massage and respiration** Begin at the pubic area and move both hands slowly upward toward your hips as you inhale. Move your hands back over the centre of your abdomen as you exhale. Repeat this for thirty seconds — the average length of a contraction in the early stages of labor.

**Superficial massage and respiration** Lie on your right side and use your left hand to massage your abdomen. Begin on the right side and work down toward the pubic area and up the left side, thus following the shape of the uterus. While your breathing is very quick, remember that your message must not follow the rythm of your breathing. Massage slowly and very gently. This massage may also be done by your husband or a nurse.

**Illust. 93**

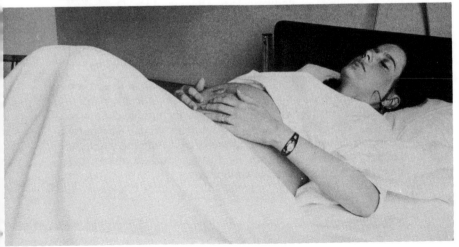

Many women having their first child experience a marked feeling of discomfort in the lower back during labor. In fact, this discomfort may be more noticeable than that in the abdomen which is occuring at the same time. This is due to the stretching of the ligaments in the lower back.

Much of the discomfort can be relieved by having your husband or the nurse apply pressure in this area. Lie on your side, with your knees drawn up. (Illust. 91) and a pillow under your thighs. Your husband places his hands on the small of your back, fingers pointing up, and applies pressure.

Do not be concerned about the pressure interfering with the uterine contractions. The thickness of the muscles in the back, combined with the bones of the pelvis will protect the uterus.

You can apply this pressure yourself by lying on your back with one or two pillows under your thighs so all heaviness is eliminated. You then press in the lower back with both hands placed on one spot, or with each hand in a fist. Breathe in with your contraction.

### The Delivery

When dilation is completed, you enter the third and final phase of labor — delivery. (See Diagram 13) The baby's head will be pushing with considerable pressure on the cervix and the doctor or nurse will now give you permission to push. Up until now you have wanted to push but have been unable to because dilation was not complete.

The expulsion is the most active phase of labor if you are not anaesthetized. You may, however, receive a local anaesthetic. The doctor will tell you when to push and how to breathe, when to push hard and when to relax. The nurse (or your husband, if he has permission to attend) will encourage you and will help by lifting your shoulders and sponging your face between contractions.

In my opinion, this is the most agreeable time, and having my husband share the experience is a positive experience which we shall never forget.

### The Mechanics of Delivery

The expulsion of the child from the birth canal is the shortest part of labor, usually lasting from thirty to sixty minutes for a woman having her first child. For a woman who has already had a child, this stage of labor may last from only five to thirty minutes.

The more supple and relaxed the muscles, the easier the delivery.

At some point during the last few weeks of pregnancy, the fetus turns a somersault thus placing his head toward the base of the pelvis. In very few cases the fetus does not turn and is born feet first. This is called a breech birth or breech presentation.

The fetus goes through three distinct phases as it moves into the proper position in preparation for delivery. Your doctor will describe these phases to you several weeks before you are expected to deliver. He will do a vaginal exploration and an external palpatation in the lower stomach area.

In the process of delivery, the child bends his head so his chin rests on his stomach. In this manner he presents the top of his head to the birth canal. The shape of the pelvis makes it necessary for the baby's head to rotate in its passage through the birth canal. As his head passes, it reaches the perineum (the muscle which extends from the vagina to the rectum).

As the baby reaches this point, you will feel a sensation of intense heat, and it is at that moment that the doctor will make a small incision in the perineum. This is called an episiotomy (Diagram 14) and is done to prevent a tear in the tissue. An incision is much easier to repair than a laceration. The incision may be made in a straight line from top to bottom (median) or from side to side (lateral) or at an angle (mediolateral). (See Diagram 14) The incision is repaired by two stitches after the delivery of the placenta and remaining afterbirth.

The child progresses toward the outside through the efforts of the uterine contractions aided by pushes by the mother. At the height of each contraction, the walls of the uterus tighten on the child, pushing him downward. The mother also pushes, breathing so that the diaphragm presses on the uterus and the abdominal muscles contract to accentuate the pressure on the child.

Remember not to close your eyes at the moment of delivery. most women do so, thinking it will help them push. However, they miss seeing the actual birth in the mirror installed overhead which allows the mother to watch.

**Diagram 14**

*EPISIOTOMY*

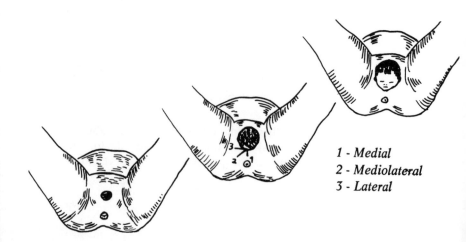

1 - *Medial*
2 - *Mediolateral*
3 - *Lateral*

A contraction begins slowly, you feel the abdomen harden — this takes from ten to twenty seconds. You take a deep breath and exhale. At the height of the contraction you will want to push but this desire will end with the contraction. This part lasts from forty to fifty seconds. You inhale deeply and hold your breath while you push and contract your abdominal muscles.

It may be difficult to hold your breath for the duration of the contraction. If so, then exhale at the end of twenty seconds or so and immediately take another deep breath. This does not affect the contraction and is preferable to holding your breath and feeling weak or faint.

If this is your first child, your doctor may want you to practise some pushing exercises at home. Lie on your back with a pillow under your head, knees bent as you breathe normally. Do not actually push while practising this exercise.

Inhale deeply and hold your breath for fifteen to twenty seconds and push at the same time contracting the abdominal muscles and leaning forward to seize your thighs or ankles. As you are in a sitting position, the effort of the push is lengthened.

Rest for two or three minutes (the time between contractions if you were actually in labor) and repeat the exercise. If you practise increasing the time you hold your breath, you will have no difficulty during the delivery.

As the baby's head begins to push through the perineum, the doctor will ask you to stop pushing for a moment until he is sure all is well. Breathe rapidly at this point, taking very short breaths. As the baby's head passes through the opening the doctor will probably tell you what he sees, as he helps the shoulders out by rotating the baby. The rest of the baby follows without difficulty.

If your husband is in the room he will encourage you as he follows the birth with great interest. You will both hear your child's first cry — a joyful experience to remember always.

The infant is then placed on your abdomen while the doctor cuts the umbilical cord. Then the child is handed to the nurse who will clean away the ambiotic liquid and sebum which covers him. The doctor attends to the delivery of the placenta and remaining materials and then repairs the episiotomy if there was one.

Successful natural childbirth is dependant upon many factors. Among these are a favourable presentation of the fetus, effective uterine contractions, good pelvic dimensions and a good execution of pushes. Only the doctor can judge these factors and it is up to him to decide whether you can remain conscious throughout labor and delivery.

When your contractions begin (usually at home) it is better for you if you walk around during the intervals between contractions. If you lie down as soon as they begin, you will have considerable discomfort in your lower back and abdomen before you are ready to deliver. Changing position and breathing in rhythm with the contraction relaxes the muscles and makes you more comfortable.

There are several exercises which you may perform to releive discomfort during the early stages of labor. These may be used at home or at the hospital.

**To relieve backache**

Stand about twelves inches from a wall, forearms leaning on the wall, head resting on your arms. (Illust. 94)

a) Tip your pelvis toward the front as you inhale, distending the abdomen

b) Tip your pelvis toward the back as you exhale, relaxing the abdominal muscles.

When your arms tire, stand leaning against the foot of the bed or, if you are at home, against the back of a chair. (Illust. 95)

Repeat the previous exercise while breathing deeply.

**Illust. 94**

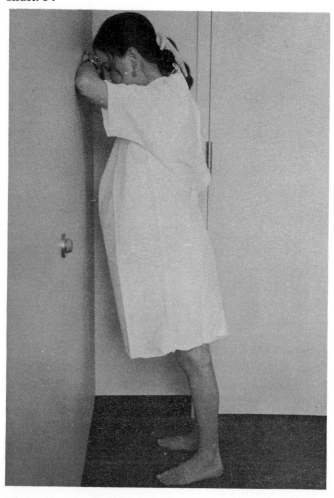

Another comfortable position which relieves backache is on your hands and knees on the bed. Strange as it may look (Illust. 96), a light forwards and backwards bouncing while breathing deeply will ease much discomfort.

**Illust. 95**

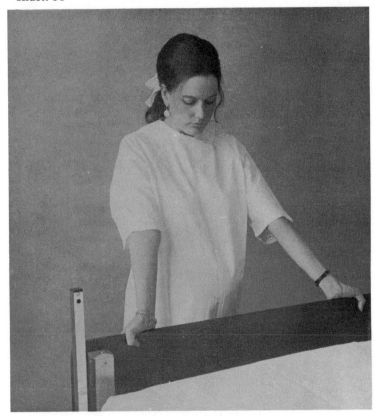

A further suggestion is to place a pillow on a table which can be adjusted to a comfortable height. Sit on the side of your bed and rest your forehead on your arms (Illust. 97) while moving your pelvis forward and backward, inhaling deeply on the forward movement and exhaling while relaxing on the backward movement. Place your feet on a low chair or footstool beside the bed.

When you want to lie quietly for awhile, have someone raise the head of the bed slightly. (Illust. 98)

If you are in the hospital, have the lower part of the bed raised and place a pillow under your thighs. This position will be comfortable for awhile, but try not to stay in it for too long because it will tire your back.

**Illust. 96**

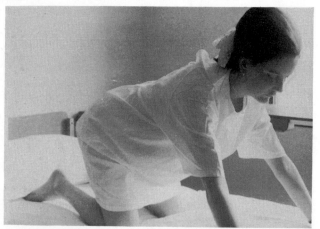

**Illust. 97**

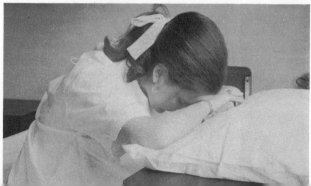

It is also comfortable to have the upper part of the bed raised with several pillows under your shoulders. (Illust. 99) You will need to have the lower part of the bed raised as well to prevent you from sliding out!

The most comfortable position for the late stages of dilation is on your back, turned slightly to the right side. (Illust. 100) The head of the bed is slightly raised and you have one pillow under your head and another under your left leg which is raised almost at right angles to your body. Your back is slightly curved.

**Illust. 98**

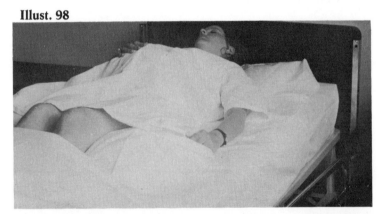

**Illust. 99**

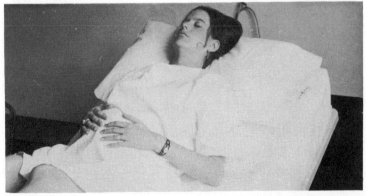

## Back Pain During Labor

The primary cause of pain in the lower back during labor is the size and weight of the uterus. From its normal weight of ½ to ¾ pounds before fertilization, the uterus expands to the point where it may weigh fifteen to twenty pounds at the end of a pregnancy. This weight pulls on the ligaments which attach the uterus to the spine and pelvis causing backache during pregnancy. However, when labor contractions begin, this pull is much stronger and there may be considerable lower back pain.

To relieve this pain, assume the position shown in Illust. 100 and ask your husband or nurse to exert pressure with the palms of the hands to the lower back region. (Illust. 101) If you breathe deeply while this is being done, you will be much more comfortable.

**Illust. 100**

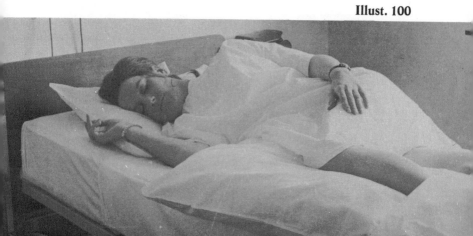

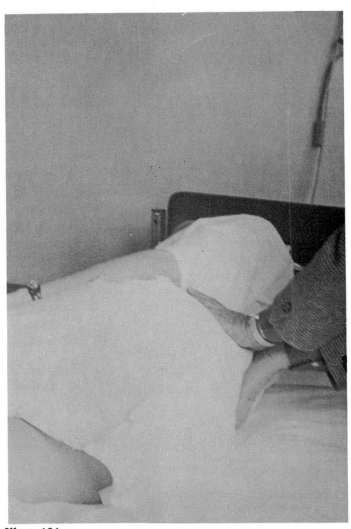

**Illust. 101**

*Dilation of the Cervix (Neck of the Uterus)*

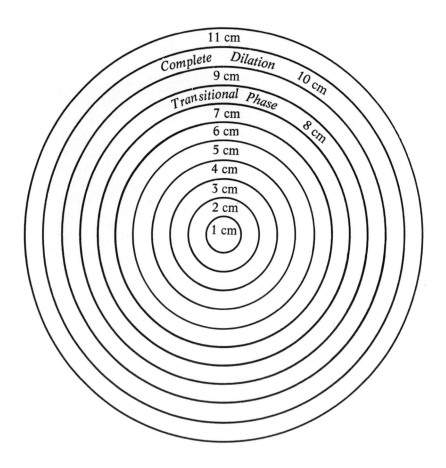

**Diagram 15**

# Chapter VII

## Post-Natal Exercises

When your baby is about two weeks old, if the weather is mild and he is suitably dressed, you can take him for a walk in his carriage.

During your walks, pay particular attention to your posture, tightening your abdominal muscles as often as possible. Do the same thing at home while doing your housework. An effective trick is to train yourself to tighten your abdominal muscles every time you walk through a doorway. You may find that you are doing this simple exercise fifty times a day.

A good exercise to do while watching television or when driving the car is to contract your abdominal muscles and hold the position for several seconds, then relax.

A good position for resting is to lie flat on your stomach, one pillow under your head, another under the abdomen. (Illust. 102) Assume this position for your afternoon nap while still in the hospital. Your uterus will return to its normal position and your abdomen will flatten more rapidly. The breasts should not be flattened, they may be painful, especially if you are nursing your baby.

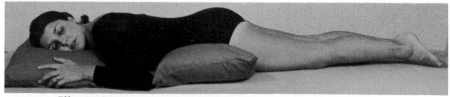

**Illust. 102**

## Post-Natal Exercises for Regaining your Figure

### Exercise 1

This exercise can be done in bed the day after delivery. It will re-establish proper circulation which has been considerably slowed down during the last two months of pregnnacy.

**Starting position**  Lie on the bed without a pillow, legs stretched out. (Illust. 103) Rotate each ankle to the right, then to the left. Repeat ten times in the morning and ten times in the evening.

### Exercise 2

**Starting position**  The same as for Exercise 1.

Point your toes toward you (Illust. 104a) and then point them as far as possible away from you. (Illust. 104b) You will feel the tension in your calves. Repeat ten times in the morning and ten times in the evening.

Repeat these exercises on the second day after delivery.

The third day after delivery, if you have not had an episiotomy (incision of the perineum during delivery), the following exercise can be added.

### Exercise 3

**Starting position**  Lie on your back without a pillow, knees bent, feet flat on the mattress, arms at your sides. (Illust. 105a)

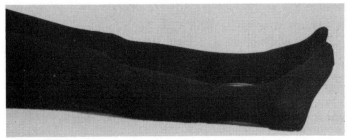

**Illust. 103**

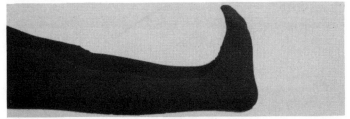

**Illust. 104a**

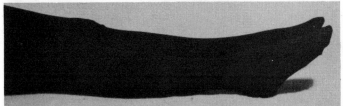

**Illust. 104b**

**Illust. 105a**

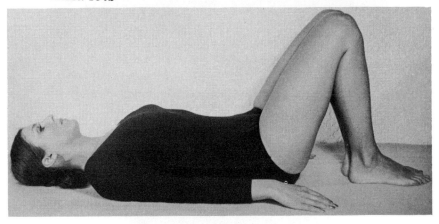

169

a) Grasp your knees with your hands, pull them to your chest while inhaling. (Illust. 105b)

b) Return to starting position while exhaling.

Repeat six times in the morning and six times at night.

On the fourth day, again if you have not had an episiotomy, the following variation of Exercise 3 can be added.

**Illust. 105b**

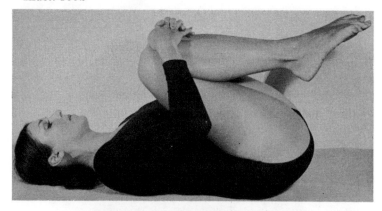

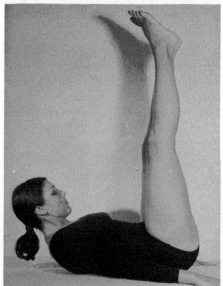

**Illust. 105c**

## Exercise 4

This is a variation of the previous exercise. The starting position is the same.

a) Bring your bent knees to your chest while inhaling.

b) Then swing your legs up vertically and raise your head slightly while exhaling. (Illust. 105c)

c) Lower your legs, placing your feet flat on the mattress, again, knees bent. Relax.

Repeat six times in the morning and six times at night.

On the fifth day, even if you have had an episiotomy, you may begin these new exercises. It is not advisable to exercise the abdominal muscles before the fifth day.

## Exercise 5

This is a contraction of the abdominal muscles designed to tone the transverse muscle of the abdominal wall.

**Starting position** Lie in bed without a pillow, legs outstretched.

a) Push out your abdomen while inhaling. (Illust. 106a)

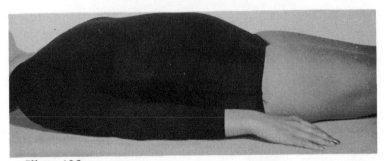

**Illust. 106a**

**Illust. 106b**

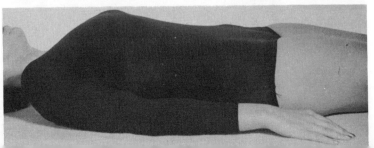

b) Contract the abdomen as much as possible while exhaling, pressing the small of the back against the mattress. (Illust. 106b)

Repeat six times in the morning and six times at night.

**Exercise 6**

These abdominal contractions tone the oblique muscles of the abdominal wall.

**Starting position**   Lie on the bed with a pillow under your head, knees bent and hands on shoulders.

a) While inhaling, swing your knees towards your right shoulder. (Illust. 107)

b) While exhaling, swing them towards your left shoulder.

Repeat six times in the morning and six times at night.

**Illust. 107**

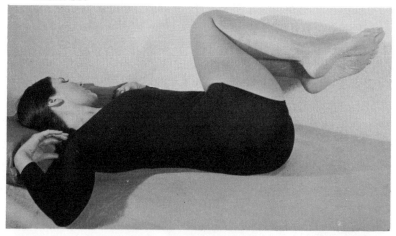

**Illust. 108**

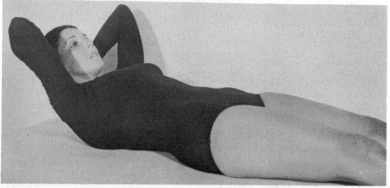

**Exercise 7**

**Starting position** Lie on your bed or on a rug, legs outstretched, hands under your neck.

a) Raise your head so that your chin touches your chest. (Illust. 108) Contract the abdominal muscles while you inhale.

b) Lower your head and relax abdominal muscles while exhaling.

Repeat six times in the morning and six times in the evening.

On the sixth day, you may add these exercises.

**Exercise 8**

**Starting position** Lie on your back, legs outstretched.

a) Raise your right leg six to eight inches from the floor. While inhaling contract your abdominal muscles.

**Illust. 109**

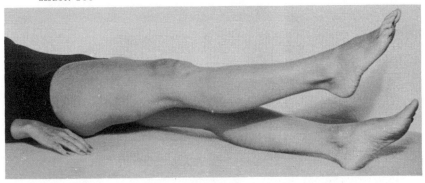

**Illust. 110**

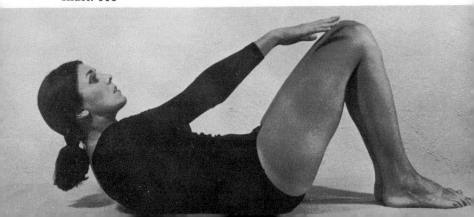

b) Lower your leg, relax and exhale.

Repeat with the left leg. Then repeat the exercise with both of your legs raised together. Stop when you feel tired.

Repeat eight times in the morning and eight times at night.

### Exercise 9

**Starting position**  Lie on your back without a pillow, knees bent, hands on your stomach.

a) Raise your head, your hands touching your knees, while inhaling. (Illust. 110)

b) Lean back and relax, while exhaling.

Repeat eight times in the morning and eight times at night.

Starting the second week after delivery, do Exercises 5 through 11 every morning and every evening.

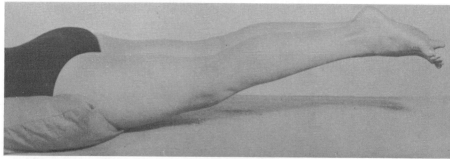

**Illust. 111**

**Illust. 112**

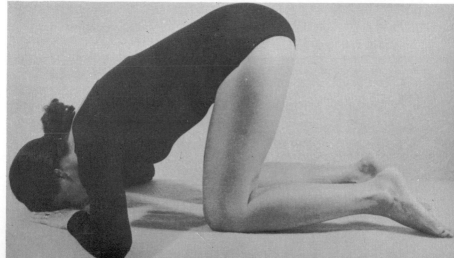

**Exercise 10**

**Starting position** Lie flat on your stomach, a pillow under your head, another under your stomach.

a) While contracting your abdominal muscles, inhale and raise both feet about six inches off the floor. (Illust. 111)

b) Lower feet while exhaling.

Repeat ten times in the morning and ten times at night.

**Exercise 11**

This exercise helps the uterus to regain its normal position.

**Starting position** Kneel on the floor and place your forearms on the floor resting your head on your hands. Place your knees twelve inches apart. (Illust. 112)

a) Contract your abdominal muscles while inhaling.

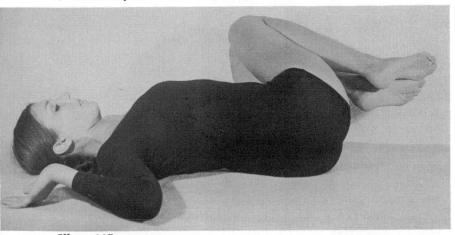

**Illust. 113a**

**Illust. 113b**

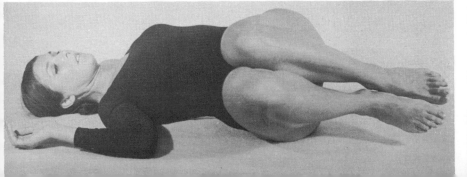

b) Hold the contraction while counting to ten, then relax, while exaling.

Try to assume this position for five minutes every morning and every evening.

During the third week after delivery continue the preceding exercises on a daily basis. You will notice that your stomach is much harder and the post-partem flow of blood has almost stopped. The next exercises will be a little more difficult, but you must continue to do them every morning and every evening if you wish to regain your figure as quickly as possible.

**Exercise 12**

This exercise will tone the abdominal and dorsal muscles.

**Starting position** Lie on your back, knees drawn up, arms bent at shoulder height.

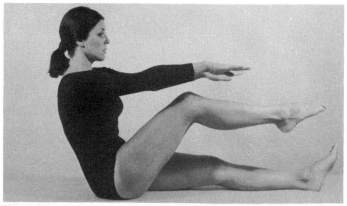

**Illust. 114**

**Illust. 115a**

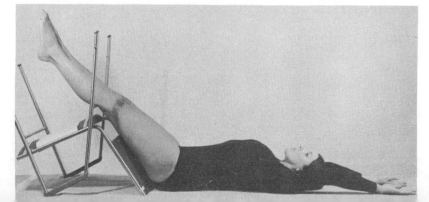

a) Swing both legs towards the left side while inhaling (Illust. 113a), and to the right side while exhaling. (Illust. 113b)

Repeat ten times in the morning and ten times at night.

**Exercise 13**

**Starting position** Lie on your back, arms above your head, legs extended.

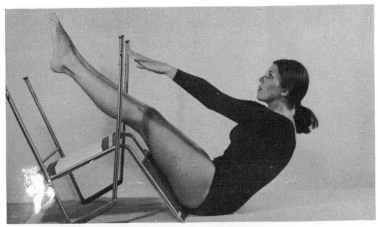

**Illust. 115b**   **Illust. 116**   **Illust. 117**

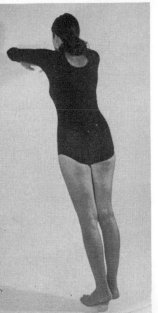
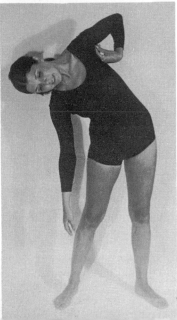

a) Raise your arms and trunk, bending your right knee towards your chest, while inhaling. (Illust. 114)

b) Stretch out again while exhaling.

Repeat with the left knee.

Repeat ten times in the morning and ten times at night.

**Exercise 14**

**Starting position** Lie on your back, legs resting on a chair or stool, both arms stretched back behind your head. (Illust. 115a)

a) Raise your trunk and arms, contracting your abdominal muscles, arms stretched out in front of you. (Illust. 115b)

b) Return to starting position while exhaling.

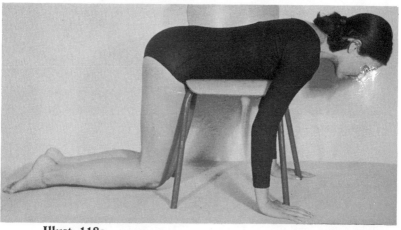

**Illust. 118a**

**Illust. 118b**

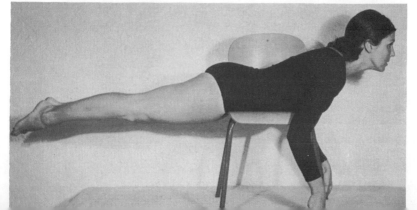

Repeat ten times in the morning and ten times at night.

The exercises for the fourth week are designed to make each part of the body work separately.

**Exercise 15**

**Starting position**  Stand three feet from a wall, feet together.

a) Contract the muscles of your abdomen and buttocks as

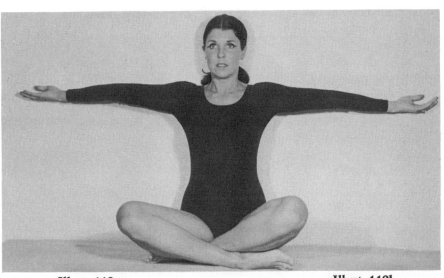

Illust. 119a                    Illust. 119b

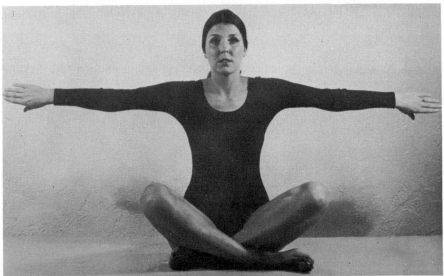

you lean towards the wall, inhaling. (Illust. 116)

b) Return to starting position, exaling.

Repeat ten times in the morning and ten times at night.

**Exercise 16**

This exercise slims the waist.

**Starting position**    Stand with your legs apart.

a) Lean to one side while inhaling, stretching down until

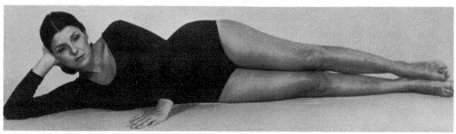

**Illust. 120a**

**Illust. 120b**

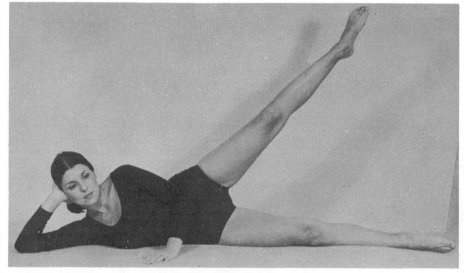

your hand is below the knee, the other arm bent until your hand is curled into your armpit. (Illust. 117)

b) Repeat on the other side, while exhaling.

Repeat ten times in the morning and ten times at night.

### Exercise 17

This helps firm the buttocks and strengthens back muscles.

**Starting position** Lie across a stool or chair so that you are pressing on your stomach and diaphragm. Hands, knees, legs and feet touch the floor. (Illust. 118a)

a) While inhaling, grasp the legs of the chair and extend your legs, pointing your toes. (Illust. 118b)

b) While exhaling, return to starting position. You will feel a very strong pull on your back during this exercise.

Repeat ten times in the morning and ten times each night.

### Exercise 18

This firms the arms and pectoral muscles.

**Starting position** Sit in the "tailor" position, arms extended at shoulder height, palms up. (Illust. 119a)

a) Make a rotating movement with your arms, extending them as far as possible backwards, while inhaling.

b) Return to the starting position, while exhaling. (Illust. 119b)

Repeat ten times in the morning and ten times at night.

### Exercise 19

This trims the waist and thighs.

**Starting position** Lie on your right side, one arm bent and supporting your head, the other in front of you, palm resting on the floor to maintain balance, legs straight. (Illust. 120a)

a) Raise your left leg vertically, while inhaling. (Illust. 120b)

b) Return to starting position while exhaling.

Repeat ten times each morning and ten times each night.

# Appendix

Here are some notes and ideas which may be helpful to you during your pregnancy and for the first few years of your baby's life.

Some space has been left for your own personal notes, questions for the doctor and a record of your visits to the doctor.

## Important Telephone Numbers

Hospital ................................. Pediatrician ..........................

Family Doctor ...................... Husband's Business ..............

Gynecologist ........................ Taxi .....................................

Obstetritian ......................... ....................................

## Weight

Normal weight ................ lbs

weight at end of

2nd month .................... lbs     6th month ...................... lbs

3rd month ...................... lbs     7th month ...................... lbs

4th month ...................... lbs     8th month ...................... lbs

5th month ...................... lbs     9th month ...................... lbs

## Dentist

1st appointment          Date .....................................

2nd appointment          Date ...................... ..............

3rd appointment          Date .......... .........................

## Pack for Hospital

### For Mother

2 or 3 pretty nightgowns
at least one robe
slippers
toothbrush and paste
cosmetics
going home outfit-remember,
you will have your figure back!

### For Baby

going home outfit
blanket

## Have at Home for Baby's Return

cradle or crib for sleeping
at least 2 dozen diapers
several blankets, depending on time of year
nightgowns
sweaters
a soft, washable toy
bassinet or some facility for bathing
mild soap for bathing
baby powder and oil
cotton swabs

This is, of course, only a minimum list and you may want
to add several items. Make sure that everything you buy is
washable. Remember, too, especially if this is your first
baby, that friends and relatives will give you gifts, so do
not buy large stocks of any item.

# Weight and Height Table

| Age | | Weight (in pounds) | Height (in inches) |
|---|---|---|---|
| Birth | Boys | 7.5 | 19.9 |
| | Girls | 7.4 | 19.8 |
| 3 months | Boys | 12.6 | 23.8 |
| | Girls | 12.4 | 23.4 |
| 6 months | Boys | 16.7 | 26.1 |
| | Girls | 16.0 | 25.7 |
| 9 months | Boys | 20.0 | 28.0 |
| | Girls | 19.2 | 27.5 |
| 12 months | Boys | 22.2 | 29.6 |
| | Girls | 21.5 | 29.2 |
| 18 months | Boys | 25.2 | 32.2 |
| | Girls | 24.5 | 31.8 |
| 2 years | Boys | 27.7 | 34.4 |
| | Girls | 27.1 | 34.1 |
| 3 years | Boys | 32.2 | 37.9 |
| | Girls | 31.8 | 37.7 |
| 4 years | Boys | 36.4 | 40.7 |
| | Girls | 36.2 | 40.6 |

# Record of Doctor's Visits

**1st visit**                      **Date** ...........................

Questions: ...............................................................

...............................................................................

...............................................................................

...............................................................................

...............................................................................

...............................................................................

Prescriptions: .........................................................

...............................................................................

Date of next appointment: .....................................


**2nd Visit**                      **Date** ...........................

Questions: ...............................................................

...............................................................................

...............................................................................

...............................................................................

...............................................................................

...............................................................................

Comments: ...............................................................

...............................................................................

Date of next appointment: .....................................

# Record of Doctor's Visits

**3rd Visit**          **Date** ...........................

Questions: .................................................................................

.................................................................................................

.................................................................................................

.................................................................................................

.................................................................................................

.................................................................................................

Comments: ................................................................................

.................................................................................................

Date of next appointment: ......................................................


**4th Visit**          **Date** ...........................

Questions: .................................................................................

.................................................................................................

.................................................................................................

.................................................................................................

.................................................................................................

.................................................................................................

Comments: ................................................................................

.................................................................................................

Date of next appointment: ......................................................

# Record of Doctor's Visits

**5th Visit**                    **Date** ...........................

Questions: .................................................................................

.................................................................................................

.................................................................................................

.................................................................................................

.................................................................................................

.................................................................................................

Comments: ..............................................................................

.................................................................................................

Date of next appointment: ...............................................


**6th Visit**                    **Date** ...........................

Questions: .................................................................................

.................................................................................................

.................................................................................................

.................................................................................................

.................................................................................................

.................................................................................................

Comments: ..............................................................................

.................................................................................................

Date of next appointment: ...............................................

# Record of Doctor's Visits

**7th Visit**                    **Date** ...........................

Questions: ................................................................................

...................................................................................................

...................................................................................................

...................................................................................................

...................................................................................................

...................................................................................................

Comments: ..............................................................................

...................................................................................................

Date of next appointment: ....................................................


**8th Visit**                    **Date** ...........................

Questions: ................................................................................

...................................................................................................

...................................................................................................

...................................................................................................

...................................................................................................

...................................................................................................

Comments: ..............................................................................

...................................................................................................

Date of next appointment: ....................................................

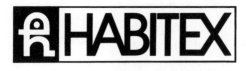

## books

*A New Series of General Trade Paperbacks by Canadian Authors Published in Canada*

**ORDER FROM OUR DISTRIBUTION & SERVICE CENTRE:**
**A.D.P. Inc.**
**955 Amherst St., Montreal 132, P. Que.**

**INQUIRIES TO:**
**Ampersand Publishing Services Inc.**
**Suite 2012, 95 Thorncliffe Pk. Dr., Toronto, Ont. M4H 1L7**

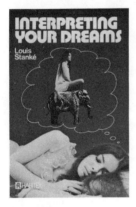

**INTERPRETING YOUR DREAMS**

*Louis Stanké*

This fascinating new book, in a dictionary format, will help the reader understand the significance of his dreams and appreciate the activity of his subconscious.

*176 pages*

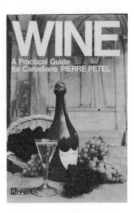

**WINE: A PRACTICAL GUIDE FOR CANADIANS**

*Pierre Petel*

A remarkable little book — humourous as well as informative — written by a Canadian for Canadians in terms of wines available in Canada today.

*176 pages, Illustrated*

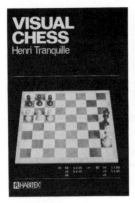

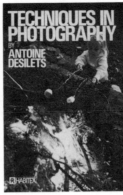

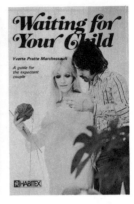

### VISUAL CHESS

*Henri Tranquille*

This book illustrates simple moves which occur in actual play and which are logical and easy to understand. Many celebrated attacks and defenses drawn from famous games are also included.

*175 pages, Illustrated in two colours*

*Antoine Desilets, Photographer Emeritus, "La Presse"*

An invaluable handbook for every one interested in photography — amateur and experienced alike.

*262 pages, Fully illustrated with photos, charts and diagrams*

### WAITING FOR YOUR CHILD

*Yvette Pratte-Marchessault*

From the first signs of pregnancy to a complete course of postnatal exercises, this straightforward and informative new book provides the answers to the many questions a new mother may ask.

*192 pages, Fully illustrated with photographs and drawings*

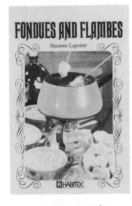

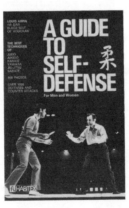

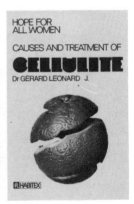

### FONDUES AND FLAMBÉS

*Suzanne Lapointe*

Easy to read format presents the recipes clearly and concisely.

*144 pages, Illustrated*

### A GUIDE TO SELF-DEFENSE

*Louis Arpin*

This book is intended for men and women who are not necessarily sportsmen or athletes, but who want to know to defend themselves in an emergency.

*304 pages, Fully illustrated*

### CELLULITE

*Dr. Gérard J. Léonard*

The author, one of the leading authorities on the subject in Canada, has written a book which will bring hope to all women who suffer from cellulite — hope founded on a scientifically based treatment which has been effective in reducing the problem.

*224 pages, Illustrated*

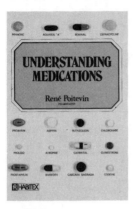

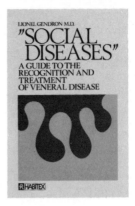

## UNDERSTANDING MEDICATIONS

*René Poitevin*

What is a stimulant, a tranquillizer, a sedative, a vitamin or an amphatamine? How do they work? What are their effects? The author, a graduate pharmacist, answers these and many other important questions.

*128 pages, Illustrated
in colour*

## "SOCIAL" DISEASES

A Guide to the Recognition and Treatment of Venereal Disease

*Dr. Lionel Gendron*

This book has been written so that the general reader may understand the causes, recognize the symptoms and appreciate the long-term effects of venereal disease.

*122 pages,
Fully illustrated*

*Printed by*
*IMPRIMERIE ELECTRA*
for
*HABITEX BOOKS*